TABLE OF CONTENTS

Introduction

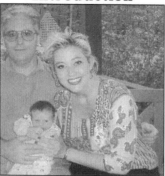

Me, before "Project Fabulous"

This was me topping out at almost 200lbs. I gained 65 pounds with my baby. There aren't many "before" pictures of me floating around because I simply wouldn't let them be taken. I was tired and achy. I didn't feel much like doing anything.

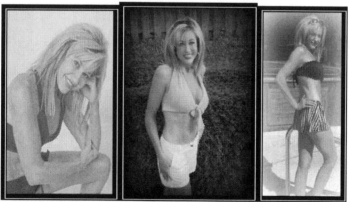

Me, NOW after "Project Fabulous".

I have learned to understand and live the principles of Now, I'm 135 lbs. and feeling wonderful!! I truly practice what I preach because the bottom line is Project Fabulous is completely "doable". There is nothing complicated or difficult about the program.

The hardest part is making the commitment to change and then BELIEVE you can do it!

4

PROJECT: Fabulous!

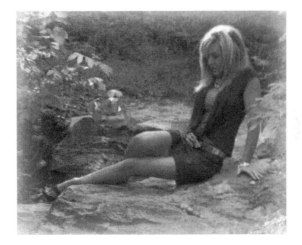

Dr. Tammy Tucker

EDITED BY
CECILIA FOY
CONTRIBUTIONS BY
DONALD TUCKER
COVER BY
EARL HALE

DEDICATION

To all those who have struggled with diet after diet... and have fought
the good battles but are losing the war, I dedicate this book to you.
To all those patients who have taught me through precious trial and
painful error what to do and what not to do I thanks you that others
can learn from your journey.

PROJECT *fabulous*

For Information about permissions to reproduce selections from this book or to purchase copies for educational, business or sales promotional use, contact:

Healthy Focus Creative
103 Somerset
Bentonville, AR 72712

First Edition

Printed in the USA
ISBN-13: 978-1463654542
ISBN-10:1463654545
Edited by: The Learning Group, Int'l, www.llcnwa.com

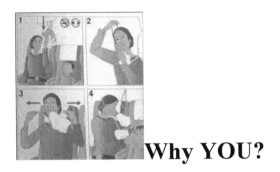

Why YOU?

Consider this...

When there is a sudden change in cabin pressure during an airline flight and the oxygen mask drops down, what are you supposed to do???

You put the mask on yourself, FIRST!

Why? Because if you don't take care of yourself first, you can't take care of or help anyone else.
If you lose consciousness you can't put the mask on your child or dependent loved one.

You have to put yourself first.

This may go against everything you think or believe, but if you are not healthy you lose your effectiveness with your children, your spouse, your work and even yourself.

Project Fabulous is about taking care of yourself so that you can take control and make a difference in the lives of everyone around you.

When you make positive changes in your life, your children will learn from your healthy choices.

Start today by choosing to be healthy and take control of your life.

ARE YOU READY?

So many of us invest years of our lives learning how to be something a doctor, artist, teacher, nurse, business executive, electrician, or any other career that you wanted to pursue.

But we spend almost no time learning HOW to be the best something we can!

How much time to actually spend developing your inner being or searching out how to be fabulous? Feeling fabulous is essential for success, productivity, creativity, innovation, relationship success, health and almost everything else in life! We usually wait for a life crisis or tragedy that forces us to look at what is really important. But is this really the best approach for change and growth?

The best approach is a proactive approach to hardwire our brains with focus, awareness, repetition and celebration.

Isn't it time to be a fabulous celebration of your changed life!

Not to mention sharing it with others on a similar journey!

Practicing the daily exercises can change the way your brain is wired.

Imagine how different you, your life, your brain - and more importantly YOUR HEART - will be when you have completed all 10 steps of Project Fabulous.

Who is the program for?

Anyone who wants to take charge of your health and wellness.

If you want to be your ideal body composition.

If you want to feel fabulous inside and out.

If you would like fabulous relationships.

If you would like to feel more connected, feel peace in your heart and feel truly alive.

This program is different from any other weight loss and wellness program you have ever experienced in the past.

Weight Loss Through
Physician Guided Hormone Balancing
By Dr. Tammy Tucker

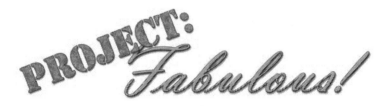

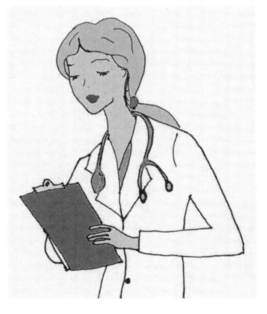

"The journey to a new YOU."

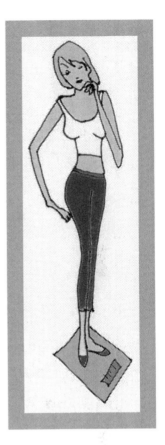

It wasn't "one thing" that got you overweight and you can't just do "one thing" to reverse it. --Dr.Tammy

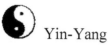
Legend:

 Yin-Yang

 Needs Prescription from you Doctor

Helpful Tip

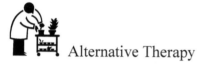 Alternative Therapy

A few words about alternative therapies:

Alternative therapies are not always benign. Some herbal therapies can interact with other medications you may be taking.

Always talk to your doctor before trying an alternative approach and be sure to tell all your doctors what alternative treatments you are using.

If you experience side effects such as nausea, vomiting, rapid heartbeat, anxiety, diarrhea or skin rashes, stop taking the herbal product and notify your doctor immediately.

Try to avoid preparations made with more than one herb because if you have a reaction you won't know which one is responsible for it. You should beware of commercial claims of what herbal products can do. Look for scientific-based sources of information and always select brands carefully. Only purchase brands that list the herb's common and scientific name, the name and address of the manufacturer, a batch and lot number, expiration date, dosage guidelines and potential side effects.

Introduction

It feels like you need a medical degree to understand all that has made you overweight.

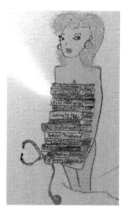

The naked truth is that you don't. You just need the ten steps in this program and a doctor willing and able to work with you on every

In this book, I will share with you all my "secrets" to a healthy new you. Project Fabulous embodies the heart and soul of what I try to instill in my patients every day (women and men) about how to look, feel and be their best.

Not "Project Barbie" or "Project Perfect", but "Project Fabulous" which is all about being the best, fabulous person they can be.

So what are Hormones?

The word hormone comes from the Greek word *hormān* meaning to "urge on" or "impulse."

Hormones are more than just estrogen. When most people think about hormones they think of estrogen and immediately fear comes to mind. Pharmaceutical companies have manipulated estrogen and made it unsafe, convinced doctors they have the only option, and created mistrust of "hormones". Amazingly, on a daily basis patients tell me their doctor put them on estrogen after having a hysterectomy and told them they didn't need progesterone because they didn't have a uterus anymore. Let me explain why this is amazing to me.

Progesterone has so many more uses than just preventing lining buildup in the uterus. It's like saying that you don't need shoes because you're not wearing any socks, but as we all know shoes have more functions than just covering up your socks. When patients tell me they are scared of hormones, I take a lot of time to undo the damage that big pharmaceutical companies have done. Their unnatural manipulation of the basic hormone structure given to women in unhealthy doses and distribution forms is not good.

We all have hormones. Some of my emphysema patients tell me they don't want to go on oxygen because they are afraid they will get addicted to it. HELLO?!!!! We are ALL addicted to oxygen! We cannot live without it! Some people need a little purer form or an increased concentration of it to help the heart and lungs work more efficiently.

Pharmaceutical companies know hormones cannot be patented. God invented them. He has the ultimate patent. By the way, you can't patent oxygen either. For marketing purposes and sales, they figured out if they changed the structure, they could patent the new compound, and sell it for a lot of money. Problem is the new compound is just different enough to cause problems. The amount is "one size fits all" and the route through the gastrointestinal tract and liver filtering creates inflammatory proteins causing all sorts of problems from joint aches to blood clots and, worse yet, cancer.

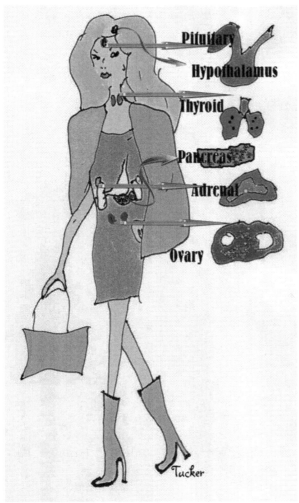

Remember, all hormones work in concert to balance each other. One is not more important than another. One may be more abundant at certain parts of the circadian rhythms, but they are always in balance.

Did you know you are a walking, talking, shopping bunch of hormones? Hormones control everything we are and do!

Estrogen – Makes us "girly"; induces puberty in females and facilitates the menstrual cycle in preparation for fertilization. Less known functions include libido, breast health and enhances female traits and characteristics.

Progesterone - Helps maintain menstrual cycle. It is more than just a hormone of uterine balance, however, because it helps with mood balance, sleep, and appetite or weight gain just to name a few of it's purposes.

FSH - Causes menstrual cycle to START. This is a great marker as a blood test if you question whether or not you are in menopause. As the ovaries start to decompensate FSH increases in the feedback loop. If your periods are irregular this will help clarify menopause.

LH - Triggers ovulation and creates corpus luteum. In guys, it triggers production of testosterone.

Insulin - Comes from the pancreas and regulates sugar or carbohydrates in the blood stream. It does this by removing sugar from the blood stream, lowering the blood sugar level and stores the glucose in various cells (usually fat). Therefore, when this hormone is elevated for long periods of time it stops working effectively and you are likely to gain weight.

Glucagon - Is produced in the pancreas and functions to raise very low blood sugar. Glucagon is also used in diagnostic testing of the stomach and other digestive organs.

Testosterone - Makes guys look like "guys." It enhances and builds muscle (anabolic). It also maintains bone density, regulates hair growth, and maintains healthy libido or sexual interest. In males, it is primarily secreted from the testes, and YES females have testosterone too! It comes from the ovaries and sometimes from the adrenal glands. Males make about ten times as much as females, although females are more sensitive to its effects.

Thyroxin - Usually abbreviated as T4. Thyroxin is a prohormone meaning that it is inactive and must be converted to triiodothyronine (T3) or the active more potent form. It does this conversion in the target tissues and works to regulate just about every physiological process in the body including but not limited to growth,

14

development, metabolism, body temperature and heart rate. It also helps as a lipid modifying agent affecting weight gain and loss.
TSH – Is released from the pituitary gland in the brain and stimulates production of thyroid hormones. It is a very sensitive blood indicator for thyroid function.

Aldosterone – Comes from the adrenal gland and regulates sodium and potassium in the kidney. It increases blood pressure by retaining sodium. It may have further indications for hearing loss and ringing in the ears.

Anti-diuretic Hormone - Regulates water retention and blood pressure.

Ghrelin - produced mainly by the lining in the stomach and cells in the pancreas and stimulates hunger. It is considered the counterpart of the hormone leptin. Highly regulated by adequate sleep.

Leptin - (Greek *leptos* meaning thin)- which is made in fat cells and induces satiation when present at higher levels. Leptin plays a key role in regulating energy intake and energy expenditure, including appetite and metabolism.

Melatonin - "hormone of darkness" released from the pineal gland in the brain when the level of light is decreased and helps induce sleep. Closely balanced with leptin and ghrelin.

And these are just a few!

Understanding Yin and Yang.

The body is constantly trying to stay in balance. The hormones are intimately connected and in constant communication with each other. They are what Chinese philosophy calls "Yin and Yang". I believe that the universe itself is bound by balance and counterbalance. Yin and Yang encompasses the all in one belief that the earth and the universe, even, are all one system. There is no superiority. Only balance. Each yields to the other without question. It takes a human mind to mess up the balance. Harmony is the balance of the system and any deviation can drastically disturb it.

We live in a society where more is better. When we accept balance, we know this cannot be true. In every decision, there are pros and cons. This is the balance that the universe maintains over us. When we accept this concept the body becomes an orchestra to be played with a conductor then we can understand how balance becomes the key issue. The concept of the universe and the moon (or lunar cycles... no coincidence that the moon takes approximately 28 days to orbit the earth and this about the time of a "normal" menstrual cycle) ties us to something even bigger than ourselves. In fact, the same root word Latin is mensus (to measure and menstrual) meaning month and echos the moons importance to measurements of time.

Also, of interesting note, every 223 months (also called a Saros cycle) the sun, moon, and moon's nodes align in the same relative angles to each other. This happens about every nine years. Then every 56 years the elliptical position of the north node of the moon moves and the sun's relative position will shift resulting in alternating solar/lunar eclipses. Is it coincidental that every nine years humans experience monumental changes? A nine year old child starts the hormonal changes that trigger puberty. An eighteen year old human starts the cycle of starting to establish societal roles. Thirty-six year old humans in our society are at the peak of child rearing and at forty-five, many humans are experiencing their "mid-life crisis". Then in our fifties, we start the cycle of menopause (yes, men do too) and then in our sixties, we start to experience significant age related disease increases and become eligible for Medicare.

So, if we deny the Yin-Yang theory and fail to realize the balance of the universe we may make many mistakes in our metabolic balance. Technologic advances have led the way to many ways we can counterbalance these lunar cycles. Pharmaceuticals now make chemicals (more on xenoestrogens and petrochemicals later) that interfere with our hormonal balances and ingest them on a daily basis.

Let me now describe a few patterns within the human body that clearly show the Yin-Yang balance.

Let's start with hormones. What comes to mind? Okay, probably estrogen. Well, if the Yin is estrogen than the Yang would be progesterone. Progesterone's role in balancing estrogen is well established and the feedback loop with one another is classic hormone science. What about insulin? If insulin is Yin, then, its Yang would be glucagon which has opposite effects but maintains the same goal of glucose metabolism and storage in body. While insulin lowers blood sugar, glucagon works to raise it.

What about the thyroid. Thyroid hormone balance (both active and inactive form) is achieved through feedback with TSH (thyroid stimulating hormone) from the brain.

Leptin and ghrelin are Yin-Yang hormones of hunger and satiety (fullness) and closely regulated by sleep.

Some hormones even have two names, like growth hormone balance. The Yang to growth hormone is the hormone somatostatin and it is also called GHIH or growth hormone-inhibiting hormone. It also has the name somatotropin release-inhibiting factor. That name alone establishes its Yin-Yang nature. Its unique properties are in its ability to regulate growth and also functions to regulate (feedback for inhibiting and releasing) many other hormones to stay in balance.

Some hormones are balanced also by the substrate or materials available within a closed system. For example, calcium concentration availability feeds back with a hormone called parathyroid hormone to keep calcium concentration balanced in the blood stream, but parathyroid hormone also has a Yang called calcitonin a hormone that lowers calcium levels in the blood.

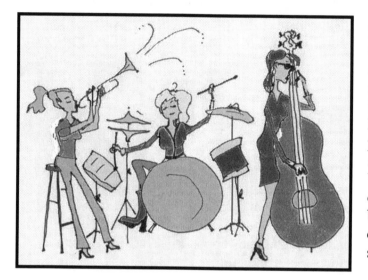

Like a fine tuned orchestra, every instrument has its own place and sound. When one is out of balance, all of the music sounds bad.

The biggest balancing act in the human body is the balance between the blood stream content and storage or usage of materials in the tissues. This balance is orchestrated starting with the HPA or hypothalamus/pituitary/adrenal axis.

The HPA (hypothalamus-pituitary-adrenal) axis is no different and drives everything you do. Every thought. Every action. Hormones are all driven very intricately by a feedback loop intertwined with one another and delicately balancing the whole body.

The conductor, in this case, is "stress" and is responsible for deciding the players and the hormones roles with each other.

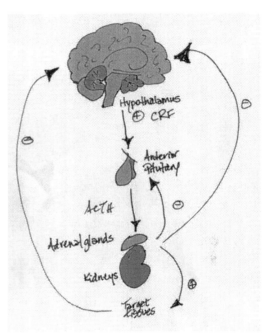

ortant key and hormones do that. There are two major classes of hormones: PPA (protein, peptides, amino acids) and steroid hormones. PPAs bind to receptors on cells and alter the behavior of the cell. Sometimes opening channels into the cell and sometimes closing them or going straight to the nucleas (powerhouse of the cell) and turns genes off and on.

Steroid hormones go into cells and exert their power there, while PPAs work from the surface to trigger a cascade of events.

Did you know you actually need your cholesterol? All steroid hormones come from the cholesterol molecule. Since steroid hormones are made from cholesterol (or a fat molecule), it can easily slip into cell membranes that are fat soluble. To keep them from just plopping into any cell they usually catch a ride on "carrier proteins", like a "hormone taxi".

Steroid hormones are further grouped into five categories depending on what receptors they bind to. These are: glucocoricoids (sugar), mineralocorticoids (electrolyte balance), androgens (think testosterone), estrogens, and progestagens. Vitamin D is a close cousin to a steroid hormone.

These are important basics because it explains why the feedback loops are so important and balance is essential, but enough with science terms.

What was the draw for you to read this book? WEIGHT LOSS gets you every time. Everyone wants a fix to their weight loss issues. When I give a talk on hormone balancing and weight loss, I usually start with something like this…

"Who in this room has ever been on a diet?" Silence. And then one woman will raise her hand. Then two… then the whole room sheepishly will raise their hands.

"Okay, who in this room has ever been on two diets?" They look around the room at each other and then reluctantly, one by one they all raise a hand.

I can't stop there. I have them captive. "What about 5 diets?" The hands are fewer and the smiles more reserved. There appears now to be a growing discomfort.

"Ten diets or more?" I ask with confidence and compassion.

"All at once?" Someone in the room will usually ask.

"Maybe?" I say. And the hands are fewer; they are just more reserved to answer.

The answer is that those who admit to being on ten diets or more are actually on the right track. They know that not "one thing" or one fad diet will work. They skip around to different diets looking for something that will be the magic fairy pixie dust they are looking for.

If you have done this, you are on the right track. The solution is simple and quite amazing. The secret is:

"All of them!"

You must be on multiple diets at one time. What do I mean by this? I mean that you must manage all the systems and hormones that regulate weight metabolism simultaneously.

"How do I do this?" you might ask. Well that's what this book is all about!!!!

Let me tell you a story. There was a lady. We'll call her Ms. T. She was skinny as a child and never really had any trouble managing her weight. College came and she put on five, maybe ten extra pounds sitting around and eating... and studying all the time. Time went by. She experienced terrible menstrual cycles, heavy and irregular. Pain doubled her over and she spent many nights in the bathroom crying and rocking from the pain. Birth control pills were prescribed and only made her feel worse. Years went on.

Infertility plagued her life as she gained a little more weight. Then, she had some abnormal pap smears and a miscarriage which was devastating to her. Finally, after many years, she got pregnant, unexpectedly. This time she carried the baby full term. Although, she was quite sick with a bout of pneumonia, she felt the pregnancy was pretty unremarkable. She had gained sixty-five more pounds and was miserable. She was still wearing her maternity clothes for months after the baby was born. Breast feeding helped drop some of the weight, but she was always hungry.

The periods resumed and were heavier than ever. She had a right side pain that sent her to the doctor for an ultrasound. The ultrasound showed she had several fibroid tumors and a mass on the right ovary. The gynecologist suspected cancer and a hysterectomy was scheduled and then completed.

After her hysterectomy, she didn't suffer from periods, but the one ovary that had been left could barely keep up. Hot flashes began and stress in her life only magnified a weak ovary and her thyroid started to fail. She was gaining more weight.

Believe it or not this lady was ME.

I am a doctor and I really had no clue how my own body really worked or how to fix it. Sure, I took biology and physiology, but no one ever told me what I really needed to know about hormones and the impact they have on the human body.

One day a patient came to my clinic, dressed professionally and quite eloquent with her words.

"Do you prescribe bioidentical hormones?" She asked matter of factly.

"Bio what?" I asked.

"You know," she paused "natural hormone therapy... like Suzanne Somers uses".

I had no idea what she was talking about, so I looked at her more intently, leaned in, and said, "Tell me more."

She proceeded to tell me about natural hormone therapy and all the benefits of it. I was astounded. My jaw dropped as she told about a world out there that was completely foreign to me. I thought hormone replacement therapy was bad, very bad. I thought it was only to be used for the woman who was soaking in sweat constantly or homicidal/suicidal.

I had received so much faulty information in medical school from pharmaceutical companies. They continue to feed us faulty information. Until that point, I believed a woman didn't need progesterone if she didn't have a uterus. I was taught there was only one way to take hormone replacement therapy and only a couple of different options or doses.

I told my patient I knew nothing about what she was talking about, and I promised her I would find out. I try to keep an open mind about alternative therapies. Many physicians don't bother with alternative therapies because there is already so much to learn and know. Why add more? These physicians ask, "If there is no evidence based research behind it (or at least that's what big pharmaceutical companies would have us believe), isn't it better to prescribe a pill?" Some doctors cattle forty or more patients through their halls a day. That doesn't leave much time to look into alternative therapies. I feel very differently about this and for this reason I vowed to look into "bioidentical hormone therapy".

I googled Suzanne and soon had unlocked a door to a world I never new existed. That was six years ago. So, what was the outcome?

Ms. T (me) started on bioidentical hormone therapy (and I prescribed it for that patient, too). I lost over sixty pounds and escaped night sweats and hot flashes! My mood was stable for once and I was sleeping again. I put testosterone in the prescription and actually got a libido back that might have saved my marriage. I felt better than I had felt since those nasty periods started when I was a teenager.

I learned that my hysterectomy was probably not necessary. The abnormal pap, fibroids, and endometriosis found at the time of my surgery were all a product of my massive hormone imbalances. I learned my heavy periods were from the excess estrogen I was storing, when I unknowingly put on an extra 10 lbs in college. From this and more, I have learned patients do not have to suffer and have unnecessary procedures, surgeries and big pharmaceutical's answer to these issues.

So my journey began. I thank that woman every day for intriguing me with something new. I didn't know it that day, but I had embarked on a journey. Looking back, this time was the beginning of "Project Fabulous".

Over the past six years, I have seen patients lose hundreds of pounds. People have transformed before my very eyes. Marriages have been healed from the ravages of hormonally imbalanced women AND men. I have been given a gift to be able to help people through this journey. I have sought out every aspect of metabolic realignment I could and this is the simplest presentation I have come up with.

The principles are really quite simple, although the nuances can be tricky. You will need a physician on your side willing to go the distance and pay attention to the details.

The goal of this book is to teach the following 10 principles and empower you to explore them in the context of your own health. It is not meant to be a replacement for medical care; rather a tool you can use to enlighten your own physician about subjects we are not taught in medical school. My main priority is you experience the three "E"s to the fullest…educate, enlighten, and empower.

Education is the first step. Explore new territories. Never stop learning. With education you can be taught, but never really enlightened. This is the next step. To truly understand what you have educated yourself about then you are truly empowered to start your journey. Healing, like life, is a journey, not a destination. I hope you enjoy the ride!

A summary of the 10 steps to your education, enlightenment and empowerment are broken down into the chapters of this book and are as follows:

- "Kiss a Pig" -- Understanding insulin and improving insulin sensitivity
- "Calories In…Calories Out" -- Controlling intake, absorption and storage of carbohydrates
- "Sleepy You is a Fat You" -- Maximizing your sleep hormones

- "Balancing Act" -- Achieving a youthful hormone balance
- "Taming the Master" -- Thyroid balance and adequate Iodine
- "Behave or Poop Your Pants" -- Tricks of dietary fat absorption control
- "If You're Happy and You Know it…" -- Normalizing brain serotonin
- "Let's Get Physical" -- Why you must increase your physical activity
- "Burn Baby Burn" -- Improving energy expenditure rate
- "It's Gotta Stick!" -- Adopting a long-term healthy eating strategy

The first step on your journey is to "Talk to Your Doctor".

You owe it to yourself to find a doctor who has the experience to take care of all of these issues. Would you let a child direct your medical care? Why would you choose someone who doesn't understand the intricate complexities of the hormonal system and how it relates to your health and well being? Once you establish a relationship with your doctor, have your doctor review your meds to make sure none of them cause weight gain.

Conditions and Medications that May Cause Weight Gain

Allergies: Antihistamines (Claritin, Allegra)

High blood pressure: Alpha blockers (Hytrin, Cardura)
Beta blockers (Betapace, Blocadren, Tenormin)
Methyldopa (Aldoment)

Contraception/ synthetic HRT: Progestins (artificial progesterone including Lo/Ovral, Ortho-Tri-Cylcen and medroxyprogesterone)

Depression: Tricyclic antidepressants (Norpramin, elavil, and Sinequan)

Diabetes: Insulin…Yes, INSULIN, Sulfonylureas (Diabinese and Glucotrol)

Epilepsy: Valproate (Depakene)

Manic-depressive illness: Lithium (Eskalith and Lithobid)SchizophreniaNeuroleptics (Zyprexa and Risperdal)

Have your doctor run some lab work or order saliva testing to check your general health and hormone levels

Know your BMR (Basal Metabolic Rate)! This is not the same as your "BMI", although, that is important, too. BMR is the amount of calories that you can consume within 24 hours to gain, maintain or lose weight. If you are reading this you probably want to lose weight. How do you do this?

There is a great program on the Internet that is absolutely free and life changing and also has an app for I-phone that is free. It works amazing, if you always have your phone nearby. The website is www.myfitnesspal.com. Create a profile for yourself and it will calculate your BMR. It will tell you how many calories you can consume in 24 hours to lose your specific weight loss goal. You have to be realistic. It won't calculate more then 2 pounds a week because more than that with a long term goal just isn't realistic. It lists every food you could ever imagine including all the items on fast food menus. You can track your weight/ progress and see how you are doing.

The BMR is the minimum calorie requirement needed to sustain daily metabolic processes in a resting individual if you did nothing all day long, but lay around. Calories are burned by bodily processes such as respiration, the pumping of blood around the body and maintenance of body temperature.

BMR is the largest factor in determining overall metabolic rate and how many calories you need to maintain, lose or gain weight. BMR is determined by a combination of genetic and environmental factors. Some people are born with faster metabolisms; some with slower metabolisms. Because men have a greater muscle mass and a lower body fat percentage, they have a higher basal metabolic rate. The lower your body fat percentage, the higher your BMR will be. The lower body fat percentage in the male body is one reason why men generally have a 10-15% faster BMR than women.

BMR goes down with age. After about 20 years, it drops about 2 percent, per decade. The more you weigh the higher your BMR will be. The greater your Body Surface Area factor, the higher your BMR. If you are tall and thin you will have a higher BMR. If you compare a tall person with a short person of equal weight, then if they both follow a diet calorie-controlled to maintain the weight of the taller person, the shorter person may gain up to 15 pounds in a year. I often tell people they are "under-tall" not overweight!

Of very important note, starvation or serious sudden calorie-reduction can dramatically reduce BMR by up to 30 percent. Restrictive low-calorie weight loss diets may cause your BMR to drop as much as 20%. Temperature outside the body also affects basal metabolic rate. Exposure to cold temperature causes an increase in the BMR. The thyroid and adrenal glands affect BMR. The more thyroid hormone the higher the BMR and increased adrenaline can increase the BMR. Physical exercise raises your BMR by building extra lean tissue. Lean tissue is more metabolically demanding than fat tissue. So you burn more calories even when sleeping.

To calculate your BMR, you can use a program on my website or many other websites have BMR calculators. First you calculate how many calories you burn in a day: your total daily energy expenditure (TDEE). TDEE is the total number of calories that your body expends in 24 hours. The average for women in the United States is 2000-2100 calories per day and the average for men is 2700-2900 per day. Caloric expenditure can vary widely and is much higher for athletes or extremely active individuals. Some professional athletes may use more than 5000 calories a day to maintain their weight.

There are several ways to calculate the BMR but manually the easiest way is to use your current total body weight

The "quick" method (based on total bodyweight) is a fast and easy method to determine calorie needs is to use total current body weight times a multiplier.

Fat loss: 12-13 calories per lb. of body weight

Maintenance: 13-18 calories per lb. of bodyweight

Weight gain: 18-19 calories per lb. of bodyweight

This is a very easy way to estimate caloric needs, but there are obvious drawbacks to this method because it doesn't take into account activity levels or body composition. Extremely active individuals may require far more calories than this formula indicates. In addition, the more lean body mass one has, the higher the TDEE will be. Because body fatness is not accounted for, this formula may greatly overestimate the caloric needs if someone has a lot of fat. For example, a lightly active 50 year old woman who weighs 235 pounds and has 34% body fat will not lose weight on 3000 calories per day (235 X 13 as per the "quick" formula for fat loss).

BMR may vary dramatically from person to person depending on genetic factors. If you know someone who claims they can eat anything they want and never gain an ounce of fat, they have inherited a naturally high BMR. BMR is lowest when you are sleeping. It is very important to note that the higher your lean body mass is, the higher your BMR will be. This is very significant if you want to lose body fat because it means that the more muscle you have, the more calories you will burn. Muscle is metabolically active tissue, and it requires a lot of energy just to sustain it. It is obvious then that one way to increase your BMR is to engage in weight training in order to increase and/or maintain lean body mass therefore weight training helps you lose body fat.

The Harris Benedict equation is a calorie formula using the factors of height, weight, age and sex to determine BMR. This makes it more accurate than determining calorie needs based on total bodyweight alone. The only variable it does not take into consideration is lean body mass. Therefore, this equation will be very accurate in all but the extremely muscular and those with a lot of fat. The benefit of factoring lean body mass into the equation is increased accuracy when your body composition leans to either end of the spectrum (very muscular or very obese).

Once you know your TDEE (maintenance level), the next step is to adjust your calories according to your primary goal. The mathematics of calorie balance is simple. To keep your weight at its current level, you should remain at your daily caloric maintenance level. To lose weight, you need to create a calorie deficit by reducing your calories slightly below your maintenance level (or keeping your calories the same and increasing your activity above your current level). To gain weight, you need to increase your calories above your maintenance level. The only difference between weight gain programs and weight loss programs is the total number of calories required.

Calories count. They are the bottom line when it comes to fat loss. If you are eating more calories than you expend, you simply will not lose fat, no matter what type of foods or food combinations you eat. Some foods do get stored as fat more easily than others, but always bear in mind that too much of anything, even "healthy food," will get stored as fat.

You cannot override the laws of thermodynamics and energy balance. You must be in a calorie deficit to burn fat. This will force your body to use stored body fat to make up for the energy deficit. There are 3500 calories in a pound of stored body fat. If you create a 3500-calorie deficit in a week through diet, exercise or a combination of both, you will lose one pound. If you create a 7000 calories deficit in a week, you will lose two pounds. The calorie deficit can be created through diet, exercise or preferably, with a combination of both. Because we already factored in the exercise deficit by using an activity multiplier, the deficit we are concerned with here is the dietary deficit.

It is well known that cutting calories too much slows down the metabolic rate, decreases thyroid output and causes loss of lean mass, so the question is how much of a deficit do you need? There definitely seems to be a specific cutoff or threshold where further reductions in calories will have detrimental effects. The most common guideline for calorie deficits for fat loss is to reduce your calories by at least 500, but not more than 1000 below your maintenance level.

It is not advisable to make any huge changes to your diet all at once. After calculating your own total daily energy expenditure and adjusting it according to your goal, if the amount is substantially higher or lower than your current intake, then you may need to adjust your calories gradually. For example, if you determine your optimal caloric intake is 1900 calories per day and you have only been eating 900 calories per day, your metabolism may be sluggish. An immediate jump to 1900 calories per day might actually cause a fat gain because your body has adapted to a lower caloric intake and the sudden jump up would create a surplus. The best approach would be to gradually increase your calories from 900 to 1900 over a period of a few weeks to allow your metabolism to speed up and adjust.

These calculations for finding your correct caloric intake are quite simplistic and are just estimates to give you a starting point. You will have to monitor your progress closely to make sure this is the proper level for you. You will know if you're at the correct level of calories by keeping track of your caloric intake, your bodyweight, and your body fat percentage. You need to observe your bodyweight and body fat percentage to see how you respond. If you don't see the results you expect, then you can adjust your caloric intake and exercise levels accordingly.

The bottom line is it's not effective to reduce calories to very low levels in order to lose fat. In fact, the more calories you consume the better, as long as a deficit is created through diet and exercise. The best approach is to reduce calories only slightly and raise your daily calorie expenditure by increasing your frequency, duration and or intensity of exercise.

Know your numbers! Know your goal. Know how many calories you can have a day to achieve it. I know, I can have 1200 calories a day to lose 2 lbs a week. I know, if I exercise 20 minutes, I can subtract 190 calories and earn some more calories. I even count things like house cleaning, the amount of energy I approximately expend during my work day, even romantic interludes burn calories and you can count those! If you don't know your numbers you will never lose the weight you desire. Starving doesn't work. You can tell yourself, "I just won't eat," but then the next meal your body will make you overeat to compensate.

Understand that the Western diet is designed to make you fail at losing weight by creating unrealistic goals of portion sizes and balance! It is cheaper to buy a hamburger at McDonalds than a salad. You must make a conscious effort to recognize this.

Two documentaries you may want to watch are titled "Food, Inc" (recommended by one of my patients), and "Killer at Large, Why Obesity is America's Greatest Threat." They both reveal the truths about our food industry. Why corn syrup has changed our world, with sodas and junk food. Why our portion sizes have changed to accommodate the obesity, not the other way around.

Restaurants give us a big plate; they must think that's an appropriate portion mentality. Did you know that a kid's meal at McDonalds can be approximately 700 calories? That's more than an adult meal should contain. The adult value meal can be over 1500 calories. That's more than most daily calorie allowances should be. Did you know that one meal at a restaurant can be up to 5000 calories, easily? You start adding them up and you will be amazed! The average adult should consume about 1200-1500 calories to sustain their current body weight.

Chapter 1

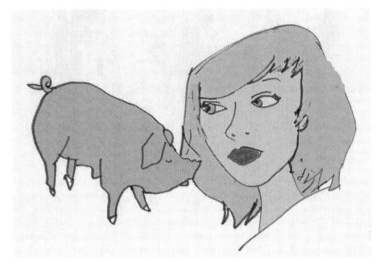

"Kiss a Pig"
Understanding Insulin and Improving Insulin Sensitivity

When I first arrived in Northwest Arkansas, I was invited to be my new employer's candidate for the Kiss a Pig Gala held for the American Diabetes Association every year. It's quite the event. My hospital marketing director, a fiery little vixen trapped in an overweight shell (which I quickly took her into the fold and made her a believer of the program), came to me one day with a sly little grin.

"Wanna kiss a pig?" She asked.

"A what?" I looked back at her quite puzzled.

"A pig." She knew that I was a "ham" for a camera (no pun intended) and eager for any publicity opportunity. She knew I had published books, had a TV show, and that my goal of moving to Northwest Arkansas was to expand my opportunities. She knew I was the person to do it. This was one of the many opportunities to share my secrets with the world, or at least the folks in Northwest Arkansas.

My marketing director continued, "Every year there is a big gala. It's the event of the year. People raise hundreds of thousands of dollars for the American Diabetes Association. It's one of their biggest money makers for the cause. So, you ready to kiss a pig?"

"Why, No." I answered. Intrigued, I asked, "So what's the pig all about?"

She looked at me with the cutest little smile and explained. "The pig is the focal point of the event. Of course, insulin was first obtained from a porcine source before it was manufactured in the lab, so as appreciation for the first source insulin they celebrate the pig.

"And the kiss?" I waited.

"Companies from all over the city elect one person from their corporation to raise funds. The representative that raises the most money through donations to the American Diabetes Association gets the privilege of kissing the pig."

So, I'm thinking a muddy, puffy, stinky thing, but she is quick to clarify. "It's a cute little pot belly pig. Someone's pet probably."

I'm feeling a little better, but still thinking about the kiss. Since, it's for a good cause, I guess, I could kiss a little pet pig.

"There's a live auction and silent auction and presentation of the donations. Some people give big items like trips, furs and cars."

Wow, this is really sounding like a challenge now. Since moving recently, I didn't know many people, but my office manager is quite spunky and I instantly thought of her helping me schmooze some folks into some big ticket items.

"Okay. I'll do it!" And off started the journey to kiss a pig.

So now that you know where the first source of insulin came from you really need to know how it affects you.

"But I'm not a diabetic!" You might be saying. Maybe you aren't and maybe you are. Maybe you are on your way to diabetes if you are not already there. I believe that everyone who is overweight is on their way to diabetes. It is a continuum of the mechanism of insulin to get sluggish and to eventually not work at all. Maybe you are on the front end. This is your chance to save yourself a lot of grief. If you have ever known a diabetic (and there's a good chance you do as nearly one in three Americans are), you know management of the disease is not much fun. There are needles, lots of needles. And giving up the foods you supposedly love? They are the very foods that got you in this mess.

The American Diabetes Association quotes the following statistics:

Under 20 years of age
- 215,000, or 0.26% of all people in this age group have diabetes
- About 1 in every 400 children and adolescents has type 1 diabetes

Age 20 years or older
- 25.6 million, or 11.3% of all people in this age group have diabetes

Age 65 years or older
- 10.9 million, or 26.9% of all people in this age group have diabetes

Men
- 13.0 million, or 11.8% of all men aged 20 years or older have diabetes

Women
- 12.6 million, or 10.8% of all women aged 20 years or older have diabetes

These are terrifying stats. I truly, personally believe this prevalence is due to high fructose corn syrup in our diets. The most abundant source is the SODA POP. A cute little bubbly drink that wakes us up and makes us feel good... is killing us. My biggest problem with the soda industry is that a soda is just a plain waste of calories. One of my mantras is "if it's not worth the calories...DON'T EAT IT!"

Did you know that an 8 oz. cola has 105 calories approximately. A 12 oz. can has 155 calories, 16 oz. has 200 calories and a 22 oz. has 280 calories!

Just to give you some perspective, there are about 200 calories in a small hot fudge sundae. I'd rather have the ice cream than the drink if I'm going to consume calories.

So that's it. Sodas are just empty calories. You are just as satisfied with water when your body adjusts to not having sodas anymore and you can save your calories for other things.

Of course, there are other more insidious reasons sodas are bad for you. They are straight carbohydrate. High fructose corn syrup was cultivated in our society because it was found to be a cheap source of sugar. The problem is that it is actually much worse for stimulating insulin production and causing weight gain. A study done by Princeton University showed high fructose corn syrup in rats with access to it were significantly fatter than those who had access to table sugar even though caloric intake was the same. They found that it leads to long term increases in body fat and raises triglycerides (sugary part of your cholesterol). Princeton psychology professor Bart Hoebel, was quoted as saying, "when rats are drinking high-fructose corn syrup at levels well below those in soda pop, they're becoming obese -- every single one, across the board. Even when rats are fed a high-fat diet, you don't see this; they don't all gain extra weight."

This new study also showed that high fructose corn syrup may be processed by the body differently. Fructose is metabolized to produce fat while glucose is processed as energy or stored as a carbohydrate in the muscles and liver. The researchers also pointed out that it is no coincidence that forty years ago approximately fifteen percent of the population was obese, now in 2011, thirty-three percent of Americans are obese.

Have you ever heard of a glucose tolerance test? If you are overweight and your doctor suspects that you may have diabetes he or she may ask you to do a test called an oral glucose tolerance test or OGTT. It measures your body's use of insulin and how effective it is at lowering the sugar content in the blood.

So, how is the test done? Well, you eat normally the week before the test. You shouldn't go crazy and should keep your carbs less than 150 -200 grams of sugar/carbs day. Then you need to fast the night before the test (nothing at all for eight to twelve hours). A fasting blood sugar is then checked first thing when you arrive. If it is normal then they give you a drink with 75 grams of carbohydrates. Then blood glucose levels are drawn at certain hourly intervals thereafter and monitored for abnormal elevations.

Okay are you ready for this? This glucose drink is just a flat cola. No fizz and no fun. A twelve ounce can of soda has 39-55 grams of carbohydrates. So think of it this way. Every time you drink a couple of cans of cola you are giving your body a glucose tolerance test!

If we are testing how quickly glucose is metabolized from the bloodstream for use by cells as an energy source, and the normal rate of glucose clearing is impaired, and we keep challenging our body in this way... well common sense tells you THAT CAN'T BE GOOD!

Hopefully, I have convinced you to give up High Fructose Corn Syrup drinks whose carb grams are designed to make you gain weight? Water is sounding better by the second, right?

So, why do I tell you all this? My hope is you have a better appreciation of insulin and carbohydrates. Since this chapter is about insulin, let me explain a little more about how insulin works.

Our natural instincts as a human are to eat and store as much as you can. Our hormones are designed to work in our favor if you know how to maximize them, but they can work against you if you don't. If you do not control insulin, then it will control you. "Insulin? I'm not diabetic." You say to yourself, "What has insulin got to do with me?"

Insulin's function is quite simple in the body. It is to lower your blood sugar/glucose by moving it from the blood vessel to somewhere else for storage. That somewhere else unfortunately leads to being overweight.

Insulin (from the word insula in Latin meaning island) is a hormone that comes from an area in the pancreas called the islets (=small island) of Langerhans. It is a peptide hormone that needs zinc to hold it together. Insulin is a powerful hormone constantly staying in balance with its yang twin glucagon. ☯

Insulin is vital to regulation of carbohydrates and storage of fat. It is responsible for making liver, muscle and fat tissue suck up carbohydrates. Carbohydrates can be many different kinds of sugars (glucose, fructose, lactose, etc.). From here on out, I will use the term sugar, glucose, and carbohydrate interchangeably. However, carbohydrates can be composed of many different sugars besides glucose. When carbohydrates are out of the blood stream and stored in tissues, they become glycogen or stored sugar.

Insulin is in constant feedback with glucagon, the hormone that signals an increase in blood sugar. If insulin has not been signaled to come out of its home, the pancreas, by elevated blood sugar levels then the body begins to use fat as an energy source for a process called gluconeogenisis that happens in the liver. Another way of saying this is the fat cell's lipids (or mobile fat...again I might use fat or lipid interchangeably like the sugar/carbohydrate thing) go to the liver to form molecules of sugar. Yes, the body can make its own sugar from materials present in storage. This is why a diabetic can wake up with an elevated blood sugar in the morning even though they have not eaten in many hours through the night. The liver gets extra busy. An important fact to understand: If you exercise on an empty stomach you are more likely to use up stored sugar than to burn the immediate source you just gave it (like a cookie).

Insulin does other things, like signal body tissues to take amino acids to make other hormones and it has anabolic, or growth effects on tissues as well. It also influences blood vessel compliance (how narrow or big they become) and brain function or cognition, particularly spoken word memory. Insulin also enhances learning. It helps to regulate temperature in response to food intake which suggests that brain insulin levels contribute to control of total body energy expenditure.

When insulin no longer signals correctly, you will become diabetic. As a consequence, you become insulin deficient and eventually you may need to take insulin through a shot as a replacement. This is usually a type 2 diabetic. Type 1 diabetics cannot make insulin at all and possibly never could.

Insulin cycles in response to blood glucose levels. There are usually three peaks during the course of twenty-four hours because, culturally, we eat three meals a day. Blood glucose may be low in the 70s when you wake up and spike up to 126 after a meal. Within a few hours, they both go back down if everything is working right and the cycle starts all over again. Ideally, if we ate five or six small carbohydrate loads/meals throughout the day, then we would never see a spike in glucose or resulting spike in insulin. The spikes and dips are responsible for overworking insulin as a hormone and making it work less effectively.

If insulin's role is to store sugar in the cells and get it out of the blood stream, then you are sure to gain some weight every time it surges. It's all about balance. This is also the reason that fasting does not work. When you do not eat for significant periods of time and your body is used to spiking and dipping then you dip even lower with your blood glucose and the body regulates up to mobilize glucose accessibility. You are doing nothing to lose matter from the system, only rearranging it in an unstable way.

Why all this talk about insulin? As I mentioned before any one who is over weight is on a continuum to insulin resistance and eventually Type 2 diabetes.

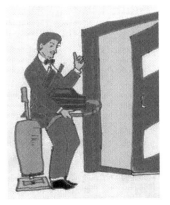

Imagine you are looking around your house and everything is pretty tidy, but there is a little dust on the floors and you realize you don't have a vacuum.

Just then the door bell rings and it is a vacuum salesman.

Great! You need one!

So, you welcome him in and he sells you a great vacuum, the biggest and fanciest one he has. You take care of the dust and two hours later the salesman comes back to your door wanting to sell you another vacuum. You, of course, already have one but he offers you a smaller handheld one. You think for a minute, "Yeah, that could be handy." And you buy the smaller handheld model.

Two hours later, the doorbell rings again. You look through the peep hole and, you guessed it, it's him again.

"I already have plenty of vacuums. Thank you." You kindly tell him and he leaves with a smile. Can't blame the guy for trying.

Just another two hours later the doorbell rings again. "Uggghh." You think to yourself. You go to the door. This time you only call through it. "I don't need any more vacuums, REALLY!" You say with a little more frustration in your voice.

He kindly leaves. But sure enough two hours later he returns. "This guy won't quit!" you say to the cat perched in the window. You think for a minute about the cat hair on the window seal and for just a second you consider another vacuum. Then you realize that's crazy and you ignore the door. After a considerable amount of time, he rings the door bell again and still you sit comfy on your couch with a good book. You think to yourself, "If I just ignore him, he surely will get the hint."

Finally he leaves. Then two hours later… guess what? He does not return. He finally got the hint. He put up a good show and really tried hard. He was successful in the beginning but the more he nagged, the more annoyed you got.

Why am I telling you this story? Because insulin is a lot like that vacuum salesman. It is successful in the beginning, but the more it is challenged, it is weakened and will become deficient. Eventually, it will not even come to the door of the cells receptors and then you are in big trouble. Now you are insulin resistant and no well meaning respectable insulin molecule is going to go to the door of that cell anymore.

Then what? Well the blood sugar is low in the beginning because the insulin is aggressive, it is ready to go in the cell like the vacuum cleaner salesman and the cell is happy to have it. After time, when you drink a lot of sodas and consume a lot of sugar, the cells do not respond to the insulin and eventually the insulin takes a hint and doesn't try to store its sugar in the cell as fat.

Elevated levels of insulin for too long can also affect your libido! Ouch. Yep. I said libido. "How?" you might ask. Well increased insulin directly causes an increase in abdominal fat which as we already know testosterone is converted to estrogen in the fat cells. This process is called aromatization and the process is known as peripheral conversion. Along with this weight gain these conversion processes use a substance from the liver called aromatase. Since the liver makes this substance, it is added demand on the liver now. The liver is needed to make binding globulins to carry testosterone around. So, if it is busy make aromatase, it certainly can't be effective at making Taxi's for the sex hormones. Of all the hormones which affect libido, insulin is the easiest to manipulate and control. A good diet along with physical exercise can lead to a healthy level of circulating level of insulin in the body.

Exercise (thirty to forty-five minutes, three to four times a week) can drastically increase your insulin sensitivity. Interestingly, when you exercise insulin levels decrease over time. If you haven't eaten a bunch of carbs before you exercise, your muscles use stored glucose since that is the only source.

This being said, if you consume a lot of carbohydrates right before you exercise, then the body will burn those and not the stored fat or carbs. You are defeating the purpose of exercise. If you exercise after having eaten, your insulin surges and your workout is essentially a bust. You only burn the calories you just consumed.

While exercise is the best way to increase your insulin sensitivity, there are other ways and those may include prescription medications. Sometimes, I will write a prescription for glucophage, a/k/a/ Metformin. "Isn't that for diabetics?" I hear quite frequently. And the answer is yes. Remember, if you are overweight, then you are on the continuum to diabetes. Metformin works by increasing the sensitivity of insulin receptors, decreasing production of glucose from the liver, and by blocking absorption of carbohydrates. Because of this fact, if you over-eat carbohydrates, you might experience the effects of the carbs going right through your gastrointestinal system. This can result in digestive discomfort and diarrhea.

Metformin is available in three different forms, Generic Metformin Hcl, Glucophage (brand name), and Glucophage XR (brand name). It comes in 500 mg or 1000 mg tablets. The usual dose is 850-1,000 mg twice daily for diabetics in insulin resistant patients I often use 250 mg twice a day or up to 500 mg three times a day. The maximum safe dose is thought to be 850 mg three times daily. To minimize GI upset or diarrhea, it's recommended you start with a low dosage and work your way up to the recommended dose.

I often put my patients on B12 injections during the course of using glucophage, as it can decrease the absorption of B12. Take a folic acid supplement to decrease homocysteine levels which may increase inflammation in the blood vessels. While on Glucophage, you should always take a high-quality multi-vitamin, as well as, extra calcium, magnesium and vitamin D.

A word about vitamin B12 deficiency:

Most people get more than enough B12 from eating meat, eggs, milk, and cheese. Normally, the vitamin is absorbed by your digestive system: your stomach and intestines. Vitamin B12 deficiency anemia usually happens when the digestive system is not able to absorb the vitamin. This can happen, if you take a medication like Metformin (=glucophage) or if you have a condition like pernicious anemia where your body destroys the cells in your stomach that help you absorb vitamin B12. Sometimes people who have had surgery to remove part of the stomach (especially gastric bypass or surgery to help you lose weight) or the last part of your small intestine, called the ileum have problems with getting enough B12. Other B12 absorption conditions include celiac disease, Chrohn's disease or abnormal infections in the intestinal system.

.

If your vitamin B12 deficiency is mild, you may not have symptoms or you may not notice them. Some people may think they are just the result of growing older. As the anemia gets worse, you may experience weakness, fatigue, or lightheadedness, pale skin, sore, red tongue or bleeding gums. You may also have nausea; lose weight, and experience diarrhea or constipation. If you are deficient for a long time or very deficient you may have damage of your nerve cells and experience numbness or tingling in your fingers or toes, poor sense of balance, depression, dementia (a loss of mental abilities).

The level of folic acid should be checked too. Some people whose vitamin B12 levels are too low also have low levels of folic acid. The two problems can cause similar symptoms. Treatment is usually regular shots of vitamin B12 in the arm or another muscle. You may get a shot every day for 1 week, then once a week for a month, and then once every month. You can learn to give yourself shots or have a family member learn how to do it.

Other alternative therapies to increase your insulin sensitivity include:

Chromium comes from a metallic element we need in micro amounts as a cofactor in regulating our blood sugar. It helps insulin transport glucose into cells where it is used for energy and helps with the metabolism of fat, carbs and protein. Two forms are commonly available as supplements: glucose-tolerance factor (GTF) chromium and chromium picolinate. Chromium can also help raise HDL ("good") cholesterol levels, and may play a role in preventing heart disease. Dietary chromium has a low absorption rate, which decreases with age, so the elderly are especially at risk. Chromium deficiency can resemble diabetes, and even mild deficiencies of chromium can produce problems in blood sugar metabolism, and contribute to other symptoms such anxiety, fatigue and can result in abnormal cholesterol levels, plaque in the arteries, growth delay and slow healing. The National Institutes of Health (NIH) recommendation is: males 19-50 years old should get 35 mcg per day; men over 50, 30 mcg; females 19-50, 25 mcg; females over 50, 20 mcg; pregnant females over 19, 30 mcg; and lactating females over 18, 45 mcg. If you have impaired glucose/insulin (you are overweight or have had low blood sugar or elevated insulin) I recommend 200-400 micrograms/day mcg a day as part of and 1000 mcg of GTF chromium a day for those with type 2 diabetes. Foods that have chromium are broccoli, brewer's yeast, grape juice, meat and whole-grain products. Some fruits, vegetables, and spices also provide chromium as well as lettuce, onions and tomatoes.

If you are taking certain medications you may be at risk for lower chromium levels. These include: antacids, corticosteroids, acid blockers, beta blockers, insulin, niacin, NSAIDS (like ibuprofen) and aspirin.

Vitamin E supplementation improves several indices of insulin action including glucose levels, total body glucose disposal, and non-oxidative glucose metabolism in both normal and diabetic subjects. Some research indicates that diabetics are low in vitamin E concentrations. I recommend 200-400 U/day.

Fish oil can reduce your risk of cardiovascular disease and lower blood pressure. It is good for regulating many hormones, blood sugar levels, insulin, and has thermogenic properties. It helps control depression, cognitive decline in the elderly and ensures healthy brain development in babies. I recommend 1000-4000 mg /day.

Magnesium regulates more than 325 enzymes in the body, the most important of which produce, transport, store and utilize energy. Many aspects of cell metabolism are regulated by magnesium. Magnesium has numerous physiological roles, among which are, the control of nerve action, the activity of the heart, neuromuscular transmission, muscular contraction, vascular tone, blood pressure and peripheral blood flow. Magnesium is needed for insulin to effectively get sugar from the blood into the cells where it's burned or stored as fuel. Without magnesium we are more prone to becoming insulin resistant.

CoQ10 exists within energy powerhouses in the cells called mitochondria. It carries electrons involved in energy metabolism and the production of adenosine triphosphate (ATP), the basic energy molecule of each cell. To effectively burn carbs as energy and not store it we need adequate CoQ10. I recommend 50-100 mg/ day (more if you are on a statin drug like *Zocor* which depletes it).

Zinc has insulin-like effects on cells, including promotion of both lipogenesis and glucose transport. I recommend 50-100 mg/day.

Conjugated linoleic acid (CLA) helps reduce fat by increasing glucose metabolism. High amounts of fiber will decrease the effects, so it is best taken on an empty stomach. In addition, it may be stimulating, so it's best taken early in the day.

Biotin improves glucose metabolism by stimulating the pancreas beta cells to work better and by accelerating glycolysis (breakdown of sugar) in the liver and pancreas. Biotin is known to regulate hepatic and pancreatic glucokinase expression at both transcriptional and translational levels and to regulate hepatic phosphoenolpyruvate carboxykinase expression at the transcriptional level (fancy talk for what happens in the cells to burn extra energy). I recommend 250 mg daily.

d-chiro-inositol is an important potential alternative to metformin. It is a form of the B vitamin inositol. D-chiro-inositol increases the action of insulin in women, decreases triglycerides, and decreases blood pressure. It's really pricey though. Some patients have similar benefits from d-pinitol, a derivative of d-chiro-inositol. It is quite a bit less expensive. And this may not really compare, because metformin is on the $4 Wal-mart list now.

Soluble plant fiber helps to combat the effects of refined, fiber-depleted carbohydrates which tend to have a high glycemic index, and thus cause a rapid increase in blood sugar. The goal is to prevent a "glucose spike" that prompts the pancreas to release insulin, which in turn signals the liver to pump more triglycerides into the bloodstream. Soluble dietary fiber slows the absorption of food, so blood sugar does not rise as rapidly, while also reducing insulin secretion. Fiber absorbs calories, as well, so you can eat more. I recommend 25-35 grams/ day.

You should strive to maintain a healthy insulin balance. When insulin is out of balance all the other hormones will be out of balance. If you are experiencing symptoms of low blood sugar (fatigue, sluggishness, cold sweats, headache) then you are having abnormal surges of insulin. These must be controlled by addressing abnormal dietary habits and considering medical or alternative therapy options.

Alpha-glucosidase inhibitors are sometimes used in the treatment of type 2 diabetes and can be used in non-diabetic individuals. One of the medications is called acarbose and improves postprandial hyperglycemia and reduces the risk of development of type 2 diabetes in patients with impaired glucose tolerance. Acarbose may prevent heart attack and cardiovascular diseases in type 2 diabetic patients. It has been shown to have improvements in glucose control, triglyceride levels, body weight, and systolic blood pressure.

As just discussed, alpha-glucosidase inhibitors interfere with the breakdown of simple carbohydrates into glucose. Alpha-amylase inhibitors, on the other hand, interfere with the breakdown of large carbohydrate molecules like starch into linked glucose polymers. These simple sugars are then broken down to glucose by the alpha-glucosidase enzyme.

One form of alpha-amylase inhibitor consists of an extract from the white kidney bean *(Phaseolus vulgaris)*. There seems to be more reduction in both simple and complex sugars by using both of these: an alpha-glucosidase and an alpha-amylase inhibitor. Such combinations are now available in dietary supplement form.

The usual dose of Acarbose is 50 mg three times a day. If your triglyceride levels are over 80 mg/dL, it is likely you should be suspected as suffering some degree of *postprandial lipemia.* As is too often observed, overweight patients usually present with fasting triglyceride readings well over 150 mg/dL, which indicates postprandial *hyperglycemia* and *lipemia* as underlying causes of their weight gain. Inhibiting carbohydrate absorption will help reduce triglyceride and glucose blood levels.

Exercise- 20 minutes aerobic activity/day improves glucose metabolism and insulin sensitivity.

Summary:

1. Cut out sodas and all high fructose corn syrup products that you possibly can.

2. Eat multiple small low carb portions throughout the day to eliminate hunger and to decrease your insulin levels.

3. Consider Glucophage and B12 supplementation.

4. Use alternative therapies to lower your insulin.

5. Use exercise as a powerful tool to control your insulin.

Chapter 2

"Calories In...Calories Out"
Controlling Intake, Absorption and Storage of Carbohydrates

Calories in/Calories out!   You have to count EVERY bite you put in your mouth. I have patients tell me all the time, "I don't eat that much." They almost plead with me that they really don't consume many calories at all. They are not being honest with me or themselves.

Maybe not intentionally, but I learned from their behavior, that I was not counting all the calories I consumed in a day. You have to count gum you chew (20 calories, unless sugarless)... You have to count that grape here or there, you have to count those little bites of this or that you take in during the day...You have to count sodas too. A coke has almost as many calories as a hot fudge sundae (regular size 150-200 calories). You have to count mints and candy, no matter how small.

Many people underestimate the calories because they want to make themselves feel better. This only creates a world of helplessness and hopelessness that will get you nowhere. Take charge now. Accept and take accountability for every calorie, no matter how small. The good news is you get to add calories back available to you in the day after you exercise by knowing how many calories you burn for different activities.

You must control your calories!

The best way to do this is to control your rate of carbohydrate absorption. Why? Because carbohydrates have 4 calories per gram. Protein has 4 calories per gram too, but is much more difficult for the body to break down. So, if you focus on decreasing carbs and increasing protein, you are "tricking" the body into working harder for you. I call this working "smarter". This is why I recommend a 3:1 protein to carbohydrate ratio.

FYI: carbs   1g= 4 cal
            protein 1g= 4 cal
            fat   1g= 9 cal
            alcohol 1g= 7 cal
            3,500 calories = 1 lbs of fat

As you see, fat contains more than twice the calories of protein and carbohydrates. Most foods contain a mixture of protein, carbs and fat. This makes the balancing act a little more difficult. Remember, calories from fat are more easily stored as fat, than are calories from carbohydrates if you burn the carbs at an appropriate rate. You'll notice alcohol has 7 calories/ gram, a good reason not to drink your calories especially in the form of alcohol.

So, what is a carbohydrate?

I still have nightmares from my organic chemistry class in college. We had to take it as a pre-med requisite. Everyone knew the teacher was fierce. If you came out with your sanity intact, you were doing well. She expected us to memorize tons of molecular structures every day. I could not possibly understand then how memorizing a bunch of sticks, circles and hexagons could possibly help me as a doctor. I just couldn't get past the similarities to "Tinker Toys". Do I use them in my daily practice? Well, no not really but I use them indirectly to understand how certain processes work and how I can help my patients through this understanding.

When you draw a carbohydrate compound formula, it still looks like sticks and circles. I find it quite interesting that all these sticks, hexagons, and circles represent clumps of molecules that are constantly sticking together, breaking apart, and when they combine in certain ways it can be the fuel that rules our bodies.

All carbohydrates are made up of units of sugar (also called saccharide units). Carbohydrates that contain only one sugar unit (monosaccharides) or two sugar units (disaccharides) are referred to as simple sugars. Simple sugars are sweet in taste and are broken down quickly in the body to release energy. Two of the most common monosaccharides are glucose and fructose. Glucose is the primary form of sugar stored in the human body for energy. Fructose is the main sugar found in most fruits.

Complex carbohydrates are long chains of simple sugar units bonded together (for this reason the complex carbohydrates are often referred to as polysaccharides).

Starch is the principal polysaccharide used by food processing plants to store glucose for later use as energy. Common sources of starch include rice, beans, wheat, corn and potatoes. When you eat starch enzymes in your saliva breaks the bonds and then the sugar can be absorbed into the blood stream. Once absorbed into the bloodstream your body distributes glucose to the areas where it is needed for energy or stores it. When it is stored, it is packaged together in a molecule called glycogen. When your body needs an "instant" source of energy, this molecule is quickly split and sent back out to be available.

If you only ate enough carbohydrate to burn immediately you would be okay. The extra carbohydrates are stored as glycogen. So how do carbs make you fat? Well, when you have plenty of glycogen for back up energy, then you start storing carbs as a substance called fatty acid which is stored as body fat. That is why carbs or sugar makes you fat as well as fat being stored in adipose (fat) cells. Therefore, although fat calories are most easily converted to fat in the body, calories from carbohydrates (oh, and protein) will also be transformed into body fat, if these calories are not expended.

Carbohydrates are an essential part of our diet along with protein, fat, and water. When I talk to patients about carbohydrates they instantly think sugar or sweeteners. Often, they do not think about the complex carbohydrates in the form of bread, cereal, rice, pasta, and other grain products. In addition, some carbohydrates are available in a variety of other foods, including fruits, vegetables, potatoes, legumes, nuts, soy, and dairy products.

Because complex carbohydrates are more difficult to break down they are the better choice for carbohydrate intake. Fiber is a complex carbohydrate that has very special properties. According to the National Cancer Institute (NCI) in Bethesda, Maryland, 25 - 35 grams (g) or 10 - 13 g/1000 calories of daily dietary fiber intake is recommended. It is important to eat a diet rich in fiber because it helps you consume fewer calories from fat and helps move extra calories in regular bowel movements.

To help you identify fiber-rich foods, select unrefined plant foods, such as whole-grain products, fruits, vegetables, and legumes. It is also recommended that our dietary fiber intake be in a ratio of 3:1 of insoluble to soluble fiber. Water-insoluble fiber (i.e., cellulose, some hemicelluloses, and lignin) is predominant in vegetables, wheat, and cereals; whereas, water-soluble fiber (i.e., pectins, gums, mucilages, and some hemicelluloses) is predominant in fruits, oats, barley, and legumes.

Consuming just 5 grams of fiber before a meal will significantly decrease your insulin levels and 35 grams of fiber a day has been shown to be helpful for weight loss. For every gram of fiber you take in, you can subtract 7 calories from your daily calorie count. Unfortunately, not all fibers are created equal. Beta-glucans (derived from oats and barley) are particularly effective as well as highly viscous fiber glucomannan.

There are some medications your doctor may prescribe to block the absorption of carbohydrates. One of these is Acarbose, also know as Precose, which is an Alpha-glucosidase inhibitor. It interferes with the breakdown of simple carbohydrates. If they aren't broken down they cannot be stored. And stored means possibly fat. Usually used in doses of 50 mg three times a day or with each meal.

If you choose an alternative medicine route with a trip to the health food store you might pick up an Alpha-amylase inhibitor. This can be found in the white kidney bean as *(Phaseolus vulgaris)* and 1,000 mg before each meal containing carbohydrates is recommended.

Avoid simple sugars and NO sodas! Simple sugars are soooooo easily broken down and just chompin' at the bit to be stored.

"Why am I gaining this weight?"

"Why is this happening to me?"

"I'm controlling my calories!"

Why is it after having taken into account your BMR and your activity level, you are still not losing weight? The answer lies in the remarkable links between hormonal balance and body fat. Before we explore these links, set aside the basic myth behind most diets — that weight control is just a matter of calorie control. That's untrue and misleading and has made a lot of people suffer unnecessarily.

The first and most basic link is between insulin metabolism and body fat. Most of us eat the conventional low-fat, high-carbohydrate diet, with lots of processed foods (pasta, breads, most snacks, beer and wine, etc.). Over time this diet commonly creates a condition known as insulin resistance. This is when your body converts every calorie it can into fat even if you're dieting. And it won't let you burn fat when you exercise.

These two links work together. Many of us combine a high-stress life with a low-fat, high-carb diet. This creates such a powerful hormonal imbalance that weight gain is almost inevitable. Yo-yo dieting, strict dieting followed by a rebound in weight, will only make matters worse because it stresses the body and damages your metabolism.

Another factor in stubborn weight gain is estrogen loss. As the estrogen production of your ovaries falls, your body turns to secondary production sites, one of which is body fat. If your body is struggling to maintain its hormonal balance, body fat becomes more valuable. Of course, if you are stressed and on a low-fat diet, your body is struggling. This is another vicious cycle.

Thyroid imbalance is another common contributor. Thyroid hormones have an intimate relationship with the other hormones in your body, including estrogen and progesterone. An imbalance in one is often associated with an imbalance in another. Because the thyroid plays a major role in orchestrating the body's metabolism, an underactive thyroid almost always leads to weight gain, no matter how much you diet or exercise.

Metabolic syndrome is a name for a group of risk factors that occur together and increase the risk for heart disease, stroke and diabetes. It is also called "Insulin resistance syndrome" and "Syndrome X".

Metabolic syndrome is becoming more and more common in the United States. Researchers are not sure whether the syndrome is due to one single cause, but all of the syndrome's risk factors are related to obesity.

Metabolic syndrome is associated with many conditions and risk factors. The two most important risk factors are extra weight around the middle of the body (central obesity-the body may be described as "apple-shaped") and insulin resistance, in which the body cannot use insulin effectively. Insulin is needed to help control the amount of sugar in the body.

Insulin helps blood sugars (glucose) enter cells. If you have insulin resistance, your body doesn't respond to insulin and blood sugar cannot get into cells. As a result, the body produces more and more insulin. Insulin and blood sugar levels rise, affecting kidney function and raising the level of blood fats, such as triglycerides.

Risk factors may be:

- Aging
- Genes that make you more likely to develop this condition (genetic predisposition)
- Hormonal changes
- Lack of exercise

According to the American Heart Association and the National Heart, Lung, and Blood Institute, metabolic syndrome is present if you have three or more of the following signs:

- Blood pressure equal to or higher than 130/85 mmHg
- Fasting blood sugar (glucose) equal to or higher than 100 mg/dL
- Large waist circumference (length around the waist):
  - Men - 40 inches or more
  - Women - 35 inches or more
- Low HDL cholesterol:
  - Men - under 40 mg/dL
  - Women - under 50 mg/dL
- Triglycerides equal to or higher than 150 mg/dL

Twenty years ago, very few practitioners were aware of metabolic syndrome. In fact, it was a controversial idea. Today, it's a diagnosis that's broadly accepted in conventional medicine. The new idea today is that there are many metabolic syndromes or a family of related disorders which lead to diabetes, as well as, to other chronic and degenerative diseases. Often times if you have the makings of metabolic disorder your doctor can use this as a diagnosis code to help you in your journey to weight loss and wellness. Obesity is a code that often does not pay well from insurance companies, so for now, this may be a way to get the insurance companies to help you with your goals instead of denying a claim because they think you are just "fat".

Under normal circumstances, our bodies break down food we eat into potential energy. That energy enters the blood stream mostly in the form of glucose. Glucose is then escorted into our cells with the help of the hormone insulin, where it becomes the fundamental fuel for all cell activity. In diabetes, our cells can't access glucose because insulin is either absent or unable to open the cell door to let it in. I mention diabetes because, it is my opinion anyone who is over weight is on the continuum to becoming a diabetic.

The following are warning signals that your body may already have type 2 diabetes:

- Increased hunger (especially in the form of carbohydrate cravings)
- Increased thirst
- Exhaustion
- Frequent urination
- Weight loss or gain
- Blurry vision
- Cuts or sores that won't heal

Type 2 diabetes manifests itself differently in each individual. And though symptoms and severity may vary, the starting point for most women is a diet high in refined sugars and carbohydrates, combined with inactivity and a family history of type 2 diabetes. Next, the body reacts to high blood sugar by producing more insulin. With persistently high insulin levels, cells eventually build up a resistance to it and stop opening their doors. This stage, known as insulin resistance, is when glucose begins to pass through the body without being absorbed.

Soon enough, the pancreas gets the message and decreases insulin production. As insulin levels drop and diet remains high in glucose, blood sugar continues to creep up. Ultimately, insulin levels drop and blood sugar jumps dramatically. This is the point where the official diagnosis of diabetes is typically made. Since the harmful effects of insulin resistance cut across all the body's systems, the severity at this point varies widely from individual to individual based on the health of their other systems. While some people with diabetes continue to make small amounts of insulin and can control their blood sugar through diet, others stop producing insulin altogether and have to rely on outside sources of insulin. Type 2 diabetes is generally diagnosed when fasting blood glucose has reached 126 mg/dL or higher (compared to a normal range blood sugar level between 70 and 99 mg/dL).

One out of three is walking around with prediabetes. Standard blood tests look at blood sugar, among other things, but leave out one of the first indicators of prediabetes: insulin. Remember that insulin levels are among the first markers of change on the pathway to diabetes. At first they increase as insulin resistance sets in, then they start to decrease. Understanding how your insulin is working can help you make important changes early on.

Sadly, many conventional practitioners lack the time to look closely at a patient's lifestyle to determine if they could benefit from an insulin test. In fact, there is no set protocol for intervention until blood sugar begins to creep up, which means the patient has passed insulin resistance already. And though you can still reverse the problem, watching your insulin levels can help you avoid type 2 diabetes, insulin imbalance and imbalance of your sex hormones.

Insulin interacts with estrogen, testosterone, DHEA and thyroid hormones. When insulin is out of balance from a poor diet, it can interrupt the balance of estrogen, testosterone and other hormones. If you change your diet, you can change your hormones. By eating balanced meals, including complex carbohydrates and high quality protein and fats, you can regulate the insulin your body releases. Getting back on track starts with making healthy choices.

Insulin control is strongly affected by the glycemic index of the foods you eat. This is a measure of how quickly insulin rises in response to the amount of glucose entering your blood stream after you eat it. Foods high in protein tend to have a lower glycemic index than carbohydrates. Simple carbs, like white flour and sugar, have a higher glycemic index than complex carbs like whole grains and fresh fruits. Simple carbs can overload your insulin receptors and make insulin resistance more likely to develop. To prevent the quick sugar surge from high glycemic foods, balance each snack and meal with a ratio of 3:1, protein or fat to carbs.

Getting regular exercise is another excellent way to help prevent you from developing type 2 diabetes. Not only does it keep your weight down, but it lowers blood sugar, helps you utilize insulin more efficiently, and keeps your cholesterol levels balanced. It improves circulation and keeps your heart and blood vessels healthy and strong. Exercise also supports nervous system health and releases positive endorphins to boost your mood and helps with depression and anxiety.

Rather than focus on the numbers, focus on the control you have over blood glucose by eating well and getting more exercise. Approximately 65% of diabetes patients die from heart disease or stroke.

We enjoy technology and modern conveniences, but keep in mind that materials used to create plastics, pesticides, household cleaners, flame retardants, rugs and furniture, electronics, and paper products contain something called endocrine disruptors which can mimic the action of hormones in our bodies. Since hormones turn on and off bodily functions, open cell doors, keep our moods stable, and so much more, it makes sense that endocrine disruptors could contribute to a shift in insulin production or utilization in the body and may contribute to the development of diabetes. There are many things you can do in your life to limit your exposure to these unwanted disrupters. Start by throwing out your plastic food containers and replacing them with glass, avoiding the use of plastic in the microwave.

Remember, always choose healthier foods. Although fast food is less expensive sometimes and more expedient than buying fresh whole foods and cooking yourself, in the long run, "Food is the cheapest medicine you can buy". And when you do need to eat in a hurry, even making different fast food choices can make a world of difference. Choose the grilled chicken instead of a cheeseburger next time. Or simply drink water, instead of soda, with your meals. Be sure to include the four food groups in all your meals. Don't forget to check the labels for trans fats and high-fructose corn syrup.

Remember, you don't have to do everything all at once. Little by little, making better food choices will help you reverse your insulin resistance within weeks.

Our cells are constantly using micronutrients in their everyday functions to produce energy and keep us thriving. Diabetes and prediabetes compromise the nutrients our bodies are able to take up, which can lead to nutritional deficiencies. Adding a high-grade multivitamin/mineral complex and supplemental omega–3 fatty acids will help fill in any nutritional gaps, regulate hormones such as insulin, and protect your body from the complications associated with insulin resistance and poor glycemic control.

It will also help your health on all levels, including your endocrine system, to limit time you spend in stressful relationships and environments. As scientists are now discovering, stress takes a heavy toll on our bodies. Ironically, the very technology invented to save us time, such as laptops, cell phones and e-mail, may afford us less time to decompress. Make time to relax and get away from the pressures of life. Even if it's just a one-day yoga retreat, a walk on the beach or an hour-long bubble bath, taking a holiday from stress is never a bad thing for your body.

Summary:

1. Insulin is a hormone that controls carbohydrate utilization. Eat small meals throughout the day to control spikes that are damaging to your weight loss goals.
2. Control the amount of calories you take in by decreasing the amount of carbs you eat in a day.
3. Keep your ratio 3:1 Protein to carbs.
4. Increase your fiber intake to 35-45 grams/day.
5. Understand that you will become diabetic if you continue on the path to weight gain due to poor choices of carbohydrate intake and abuse of your pancreas in the production of insulin.

Chapter 3

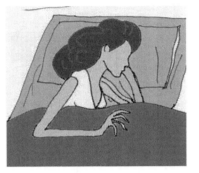

"A Sleepy You is a Fat You"
Maximizing Your Sleep Hormones

Researchers say that how much you sleep and how well you sleep may silently orchestrate a symphony of hormonal activity tied to your appetite. According to the National Sleep Foundation, the average woman gets only six and a half hours of sleep per night. Chronic sleep deprivation can have a variety of effects on the metabolism and overall health.

You've heard it before. "Gotta get your beauty sleep". It's really true. If you don't get adequate sleep you will have a very difficult time losing weight. The main reason is that when you don't get enough sleep a hormone called Ghrelin is released in excess. Ghrelin is a hormone that is known to stimulate appetite. Leptin is the yang of Ghrelin.

Leptin is known to decrease appetite and is abundant when sleep is adequate. Usually this is around 8-9 hours for the average adult. In 2006 at the American Thoracic Society International Conference, it was shown that women who slept 5 hours per night were 32% more likely to experience major weight gain (an increase of 33 pounds or more) and 15% more likely to become obese over the course of the 16-year study, compared to those who slept 7 hours a night. Those women who slept 6 hours per night were still 12% more likely to experience major weight gain and are 6% more likely to become obese, compared to women who slept 7 hours a night.

Just a few days of sleep restriction starts an abnormal cascade of hormone imbalances that increase hunger. Even if you eat less, you will still gain weight. Then, there is the impact of cortisol levels. When you don't get enough sleep, there is an increase in cortisol that also stimulates hunger, affects insulin and may therefore add to unwanted weight gain. It does this by decreasing the ability to process carbohydrates, manage stress, and maintain a proper balance of hormones. In just one sleep-restricted week, research study participants had a significant loss in their ability to process glucose and had an accompanying rise in insulin.

Your basal metabolic rate thermostat (calories you burn at rest) may be reset when you do not receive adequate sleep in a negative way. Also, those that don't rest well are tired and may not move around as much during the day to burn calories. Inadequate sleep can reduce levels of growth hormone that regulate the body's proportions of fat and muscle, so not only are you fat, but you'll be "lumpy".

As mentioned, sleep quality is important to assess as well. The hit show "The Biggest Loser" knows this, too. Since the show's seventh season, sleep studies have been added to the contestants' pre-show medical work-ups. Those with sleep apnea receive treatment. Doctors found that a majority of the contestants had sleep apnea, not surprising a neck measurement of 17 inches puts you at great risk, and often severe cases. In one season, every cast member had a positive sleep apnea diagnosis according to the National Sleep Foundation's website. This website has an interesting interview of Sean Algaier and how sleep apnea affected his life.

The Greek word "apnea" literally means "without breath." There are three types of apnea: obstructive, central, and mixed. Of the three, obstructive is the most common. Despite the difference in the root cause of each type in all three, people with untreated sleep apnea stop breathing repeatedly during their sleep, sometimes hundreds of times during the night and often for a minute or longer.

Snoring is not normal. It runs the emotional gambit of cute to down right annoying to most. Marriages have ended over it. Some people think that it is okay to snore. It isn't. The sound of the snore is from a physical blockage of the airway or obstruction. Obstructive sleep apnea (OSA) is caused usually when the soft tissue in the rear of the throat collapses and closes during sleep. In central sleep apnea, the brain fails to signal the muscles to breathe. Mixed apnea, as the name implies, is a combination of the two. With each apnea event, the brain briefly arouses people with sleep apnea in order for them to resume breathing, but consequently sleep is extremely fragmented and of poor quality.

Sleep apnea is very common.

Risk factors include being male, overweight, and over the age of forty. It can affect anyone of any age, even kids. There seems to be an insurmountable lack of awareness by the public and healthcare professionals. The vast majority remain undiagnosed and therefore untreated, despite the fact that this serious disorder can have significant consequences like high blood pressure, congestive heart failure, impotency, weight gain and headaches. Something else scary is that untreated sleep apnea could cause accidents at work or car wrecks from being sleep deprived and sleepy during the day. Fortunately, sleep apnea can be diagnosed and treated. Several treatment options exist. Sometimes, this is in the form of a mask called a cpap that holds the airway open, surgery to remove extra tissues, and even sewing a tennis ball to your pajama back to prevent you from rolling onto your back.

Which came first, "The chicken or the egg?"... I sometimes wonder if obesity causes sleep apnea or if sleep apnea causes obesity. Either way it should always be addressed in any weight loss program.

Some people have a hard time going or staying asleep. You may need to address something called sleep hygiene.
These are regular patterns that may assist you in going or falling asleep and include:

Use the bedroom for sleep only. Don't use the bedroom as an office or for watching TV before bed. You want to reduce any stimulation when you are trying to wind down. One of the biggest mistakes people make in corrupting their sleep is to use their bedroom for activities other than sleep or sex.

You should establish regular sleeping and waking times. Brain confusion can occur and shift workers have a really hard time with this issue.

Have a bedtime routine like showering or washing your face, prayer, meditation, reading or deep breathing and relaxation.

Avoid spicy food, caffeine, sugar and alcohol (Alcohol is initially sedating but causes CNS excitation later) at least 4 to 6 hours prior to going to sleep.

Develop a regular exercise program. Exercise and good nutrition will help enhance sleeping patterns. However, avoid exercising 2 hours before sleeping, since this may stimulate your body and make sleeping more difficult.

Block out distracting noises and lights. You are in your bedroom to sleep and not to be distracted by environmental interferences. Melatonin is a hormone that promotes sleep and is increased when the room is really dark.

You may want to keep a sleep log that details your sleeping patterns, habits and improvements. This can be used and reviewed each time you find yourself with disrupted sleep patterns.

Limit nicotine exposure.

Limit liquids after 8pm to avoid getting up to urinate.

Drink a calming herbal tea such as chamomile or peppermint, unless urinating at night is an issue.

Do not take your worries to bed - write them down and set aside a designated time to deal with them.

Use comfortable bedding

Sleep in a well-ventilated room that is neither too hot nor too cold. (A cooler room is better.)

Avoid pets sleeping in the bed with you as they may interfere with a full night's sleep. Consider keeping them on the floor.

Talk to your doctor if you are having trouble with sleep. Make sure that they order appropriate tests to assess for sleep problems. There are medications to aid with sleep, but oftentimes, getting your body's hormones in balance is all that you need.

Some alternative therapies that may help with sleep:

Herbs: Valerian Root (*Valeriana officinalis*), Chamomile, passionflower, hops, ginsing, lemon balm and skullcap.

Melatonin: Melatonin is a hormone that plays a critical role in the regulation of sleep-wake cycle and other circadian rhythms.

Melatonin has been studied as a possible treatment of circadian rhythm disorders and jet lag. I usually recommend 3-9 mg at bedtime.

Acupuncture: Traditional Chinese Medical (TCM) requires that the underlying pattern of disharmony be defined in each case of insomnia and treated accordingly. Most classical texts describe 4-6 underlying patterns that result in sleep problems. Each is defined by a landscape of symptoms and then the acupuncturist uses many different tools to confirm the clinical impression. Insomnia is thought to be that the Shen is disturbed, due to either insufficient tranquility (deficient yin energy) or excess stimulation (yang energy). Manifestations of Shen disturbance include palpitations, dizziness and most commonly insomnia. It is thought that if you awaken at the same time every night that the body's life force energy (Qi) flows through the different meridians at a specific time of day and spends 2 hours in each one. Thus, if a person complains he/she awakens at the same hour each night, insight is gained into the nature of the disharmony. Acupuncture and Chinese herbs are excellent treatment options to correct these underlying disharmonies. An acupuncturist may also recommend nutritional supplements and homeopathic remedies to address underlying causes of sleep disturbance.

Relaxation, meditation, guided imagery, hypnosis or massage: Increased muscle tension and intrusive thoughts interfere with sleep. Progressive muscle relaxation and biofeedback and quieting the mind with meditation may help. Yoga practice may result in higher blood levels of melatonin, too. Recent studies show that even the low-to-moderate Tai Chi and Tibetan Yoga practices enhance sleep quality.

Aromatherapy: Aromatherapy is the therapeutic use of essential oils to comfort and heal or promote wellness. The essential oils are used topically rather than taken internally. The essential oils are said to stimulate an area of the brain, known as the limbic system that controls mood and emotion. Many people find it a soothing complement to other self-help measures to ease tension, promote relaxation, and aid in sleep as part of their bedtime preparations. So, you may want to give it a try.

The essential oils are generally available at health food stores, although these days many drugstores also carry a variety of the oils. The most commonly recommended oil for promoting sleep is lavender. There are several others that may have a calming effect and you may want to combine different oils to enhance the effect. You can add a few drops to a warm bath or spritz the oil in a small pillow or piece of fabric or use a diffuser. You can use an unscented "carrier" oil like grape seed or almond oil and add a few drops of the essential oil for a combined effect of massage and aromatherapy.

Regular exercise: deepens sleep in young adults with or without sleep disorders. In addition, several studies show that exercise can improve sleep in older adults.

Prescription medication that may help with sleep:

Antidepressants like Trazadone or Elavil (Caution. These can contribute to weight gain). Rozerem, also known, as Ramelteon which is in a class of medications called melatonin receptor agonists. It works similarly to melatonin,

Prescription sleep medications are generally sedative-hypnotics; most, but not all, are barbiturates and benzodiazepines. Benzodiazepines, a family that includes Valium®, Xanax®, Ativan®, Halcion®, Dalmane® , Restoril®, Tranxene®, Klonopin® and Librium®.

Sedative-hypnotics are central nervous system depressants. They work by increasing the activity of GABA (Gamma Amino Butyric Acid), the principal neurotransmitter in the brain for CNS depression. Sedative-hypnotic medications mask the symptoms of insomnia, but are not curative. When the medication is discontinued, the symptoms of the sleep problem will probably resume. Worse still, since sedative-hypnotics can be habit forming, they can dangerous to use over a prolonged period of time. Patients can even develop addictions to sleep medication. In these instances ever-greater amounts of medication are needed to get a therapeutic effect as tolerance develops. Patients can suffer a withdrawal syndrome similar to that found in alcoholism if they abruptly discontinue the drug. Rebound effects from the discontinuation of sedative-hypnotics, ironically, include insomnia and irritability. These should only be used short term, if at all. Over the counter sleep aids are usually antihistamines that cause drowsiness (such as, Nytol, Sleep-Eez and Sominex) or a combination of an antihistamine and a pain reliever (Anacin P.M., Excedrin P.M., and Tylenol P.M). They can help with sedation but are not a good long term solution as they may have side effects and daytime drowsiness or "hangover" can be an issue.

Summary:

Get at least 8 hours of sleep a night to increase your body's ability to keep your metabolism and appetite hormones in check.

Sleep quality is important too. If you have risk factors for sleep apnea or symptoms ask your doctor for further tests.

If you have trouble going or staying asleep, assess your sleep hygiene.

Ask your doctor about different choices for temporary sleep-aids if you need them.

Chapter 4

"Balancing Act"
Achieving a Youthful Hormone Balance

So often, I have patients tell me they had their steroid hormone levels checked and they were told they were "fine". My first response is, "If you are 'fine', then why are you having symptoms?" My next question is what reference range were they using? An estrogen level in a little girl is much different than an adult female. An adult menstruating female has different hormone levels than a postmenopausal lady, right? So many times women tell me their doctor said they were in menopause so "of course their hormone levels are low"; like it's normal. But, I assure you it isn't. If you want to feel like you are in your twenties or thirties, you can't have the hormone levels of a sixty or seventy year old female.

What is normal really? If you have ever seen a range of averages plotted out on a bell curve you know that you can be on the low end or the high end and still be part of the curve. But if you are having symptoms and on one extreme end of the bell curve or the other then are you really normal and maybe your body operates at a higher level maximally but this will not be reflected on an averages curve. We know that levels that are normal in your youth may not be levels that are present after organs like your ovaries fail. So it may be normal not to have much sex steroid hormone around after menopause, according to the numbers game, but does that mean that you will feel like you did when the levels were higher? Probably not.

You are smarter than that. You are proactive and we are all looking for the fountain of youth. Well, it may not be magical or overnight, but we can restore balance and feel better.

When we think about youthful hormones the steroid or sex hormones are first and foremost. Why? Because when you are at the time in your life when you peak sexually it is the time you feel the best.

Generally, the steroid hormones come from the reproductive organs. In females these are the ovaries; and in males these are the testes. The body has an amazing ability to secure back up plans and the back up production of these hormones is from the adrenal glands. These little organs sit on top of your kidneys and produce stress hormones and hormones of your fluid and electrolyte balance. It is because of the adrenals production of sex/steroid hormones that you have any sex hormones after menopause.

The steroid hormones are grouped into five main categories by the receptors that they bind to. These are glucocorticoids, mineralocorticoids, androgens (testosterone), estrogens, and progestagens.

From a simplistic point of view, each of these hormones produces certain effects. Some of them you can see, like hair growth or a menstrual cycle. Some you can't see, like internal balance mechanisms.

Oftentimes, I tell women in my practice, I know what they need to adjust based on the symptoms they tell me they are having more than a blood test will ever tell me.

What are designer "bio-identical hormones?

They are the hormones that are identical to the human body's hormones. When the word 'designer' is brought in for discussion, we are talking about the fact that one size does not fit all. The doses are tailored to our individual needs. People need different clothes sizes; our human hormones can vary quite a bit. Even environments affect our hormones through different levels of stress.

The questionnaire I have my patients fill out is a quite lengthy, but it helps me to understand them better and how to dose their hormone replacement adequately.

To help you assess the severity of your hormone imbalance addressing the following list of symptoms or issues may help you monitor and keep track of your hormone balance. I have patients check the box if they are having symptoms and then record Mild, Moderate, or Severe after the response.

[] PMS(premenstrual syndrome) issues… cramps, nausea, breast tenderness, headaches, and/or irritability 1-2 weeks before my period

[] Difficulty falling asleep or staying asleep

[] Fatigue or loss of energy especially in the afternoon

[] Frequent bouts of irritability and depression

[] Frequent anxious feelings, anxiety attacks, or heart palpitations

[] Achy or stiff joints, especially in the morning

[] Gaining weight, especially around the middle

[] Losing weight is more difficult than in the past

[] Pain with intercourse

[] Inability to have orgasm, decreased sensitivity, or decreased sex drive

[] Vaginal dryness

[] Crave sweets, carbohydrates or alcohol.

[] Hair or skin that is dry, fragile, or thinning

[] Losing inches of height, diagnosed with osteoporosis, suffered from broken or fractured bones.

[] Recurrent yeast or urinary tract infections.

[] Irregular menstrual periods.

[] Hot flashes or night sweats.

[] Missing the outer third of your eyebrows

[] Frequent headaches or migraines

[] Fluid retention (rings fit tight or shoe size increased)

[] History of cysts on ovaries

[] Male distribution hair growth (facial hair, male pattern balding)

[] Problems with acne or rosacea

[] Heart racing or irregular heart beats felt

[] Hot or cold intolerance

[] Constipation or diarrhea

[] Frequent bouts of abdominal bloating or gas

[] Skin rashes or new onset allergies

Bioidentical hormones are manufactured in the lab to have the same molecular structure as the hormones made by your own body. By contrast, synthetic hormones are intentionally different. Drug companies can't patent a bioidentical structure, so they invent synthetic hormones that are patentable.

It's so unbelievable to me that bioidentical hormones have been around for years, although most doctors have never heard of them. Big pharmaceutical companies who have expensive patented synthetic hormones would like to make sure they never do. The biggest problem is that one size does not fit all when it comes to hormone therapy and most of the traditional synthetic hormone therapies are only that. One or two, maybe three different doses.

By contrast, the bioidentical or designer hormones are dosed specifically to a patient's blood or saliva hormone levels but mostly by symptoms or concerns. It's important to have your doctor order lab tests (saliva or blood) to establish baselines, rule out serious disease/tumors, and to assess success of absorption into the system from time to time. Not every person needs hormone therapy. When they do though, many medical studies suggest that bioidentical hormones are safer than synthetic versions. It is often possible to rebalance hormones without the use of hormonal supplementation by using nutritional supplements, gentle endocrine support, and dietary and lifestyle changes.

Even with this foundation, a minority of women will need to add prescription-strength hormone supplements to get complete relief, at least through a transition period. We recommend they use bioidentical hormones, preferably in a compounded form personalized to their needs by an experienced practitioner.

There is no substance we introduce into our bodies that is not without potential side effects. Even water can be dangerous when you drink too much. There has been a lot of press around the negative statements from the WHI (women's health initiative) studies on the effectiveness and health risks of HRT, but it is important to remember that these studies were based on synthetic/equine-based hormones that were taken by mouth.

The WHI was launched in 1991 and consisted of a set of clinical trials and an observational study, which together involved 161,808 generally healthy postmenopausal women. The clinical trials were designed to test the effects of postmenopausal hormone therapy, diet modification, and calcium and vitamin D supplements on heart disease, fractures, and breast and colorectal cancer. The hormone trial had two studies: the estrogen-plus-progestin study of women with a uterus and the estrogen-alone study of women without a uterus. In both hormone therapy studies, women were randomly assigned to either the hormone medication being studied or to placebo.

I personally feel the benefits of bioidentical natural hormone therapy are more than just symptom relief. I rarely run into a woman who is not symptomatic from some sort of hormonal imbalance symptoms; regardless, I feel the benefits of preventing osteoporosis and keeping the mind, skin and blood vessels youthful is of upmost importance.

With all the controversy around hormones and breast cancer, the question comes up, "What about bioidentical hormones if a person has had breast cancer?"

The pendulum has swung so far that very few doctors will prescribe any type of HRT, synthetic or bioidentical, for women who have had breast cancer or even a family history of breast cancer. There may still be options for you if you are at higher risk. If you are interested in learning more about this here is a great website:
http://www.project-aware.org/Resource/articlearchives/hrt-breastcancer.shtml

I recommend you read Dr. John Lee's book, "What your doctor may not tell you about breast cancer". He also has several other great books that I consider to be my "bibles" of hormone education study.

Not all estrogens are alike…..

Estrogen often gets a "bad rap" because of synthetic versions.

Premenopausal women produce three biologically active estrogens, estrone (E1), estradiol (E2), and estriol (E3). Estradiol is the most abundant estrogen produced and both estrone and estradiol are potent estrogens. Estriol is considered a weak estrogen. Although little scientific data supports the claim, it has been postulated that estrone is a "bad" estrogen and may be the cause of estrogen's cancer-causing properties, while estriol is a "good" estrogen and may protect against cancer. Estradiol is probably neutral.

Oral estrogens, not estrogens given by systemic routes (patch, skin cream, vaginal cream, under the tongue), are converted into estrone with potential negative effects for the patient. Oral estrogens, because they are metabolized by the liver, likely exert different effects than systemic estrogens which are not metabolized by the liver.

So, yes, women who have had breast cancer might consider this alternative if they are symptomatic with menopause or pre-menopause. It is thought estrone is a "bad" estrogen and may be the cause of estrogen's cancer-causing properties. Estradiol is probably neutral, but helps significantly with hot flashes.

Over 13 million women were on some form of synthetic HRT before the initial studies were published. When the studies came out millions quit "cold turkey". I can only imagine all those women and their symptoms returning. Many stayed on synthetic HRT, but live in fear of the consequences and hormone replacement therapy side effects. Many of those women were unnecessarily placed on antidepressants as pharmaceutical companies and doctors gained alliance to position those drugs as substitute products for lack of hormone balance. Most of these women were not depressed and now have been exposed to a new set of potential side effects.

The majority of studies published to date have concerned synthetic HRT, specifically Premarin and Prempro. Both of these forms are usually take in pill form or orally. Studies have shown levels of CRP (c-reactive protein) are increased with intake of oral estrogen. CRP is a pro-inflammatory blood protein associated with increased risk of heart attack and stroke. Very few have involved or reported anything about bioidentical hormone replacement therapy. Oral estrogens are converted into estrone with potential negative effects; not estrogens given by transdermal or through the skin routes (patch, skin cream, vaginal cream, under the tongue).

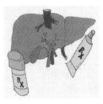

Why Creams and gels?

Oral hormones, with a focus on estrogen, are metabolized by the liver. This is known as first pass metabolism. When this happens a normal process occurs that creates "inflammatory proteins". These proteins can cause many different types of inflammation in the body. Of most concern are the blood vessels with a risk of a heart attack or a stroke.

When a route through the skin is chosen, this first pass metabolism by the liver is bypassed and goes straight to the tissues that need it.

This is why we choose creams and gels.

Although I do not recommend oral estrogen, there were problems with the WHI study that no one really talks about. For one thing, the women in the WHI studies were on HRT after menopause while the most common therapeutic use of HRT is for perimenopausal symptoms. Also, the higher risks are small in absolute terms, the increases in relative risk are significant. To take heart attack as one example, the WHI data taken as a whole indicated that out of 10,000 women on Prempro, an extra six would have a heart attack each year compared to women not on Prempro. That may not seem like a substantial risk, but it is a much greater relative risk. The WHI study indicated that the overall increase for women on Prempro for breast cancer was 26%, for heart attack 29%, for stroke 41%, for blood clots 100%, and for Alzheimer's or dementia over 100%. Many of the top problems in women's health are on that list. And, even if, there is not as great a risk of heart attack as originally supposed, for women closer to menopause, the overall risk-benefit ratio is significant.

Thankfully, there are good alternatives to synthetic HRT. Dr. John Lee, author of *What Your Doctor May Not Tell You About*

Menopause, a pioneer of bioidentical hormone therapy stated that there are three rules to hormone replacement therapy. The first rule is to use hormones only if you "need" them (based on lab values or symptoms). The second rule is to use bioidentical hormones and never synthetic, and the third rule is to only use hormone replacement in dosages that create hormone balance. Many women don't even require hormone therapy. Sometimes symptoms can be controlled by a program of core nutritional and endocrine support.

Many women who switch over from oral synthetic estrogen to natural forms of estrogen and progesterone undergo a transition period. It is as if the body's hormone receptors have been primed by the synthetic molecules and have trouble recognizing other forms, even a woman's own. Sometimes, the transition can take four to six weeks. I often start slowly reducing the synthetic dose (not quitting cold turkey from the oral form) as I start with a low dose of bioidentical estrogen and titrate up slowly as the synthetic is getting out of the system. If you stop too abruptly, you may experience extreme hot flashes or other symptoms may flare due to the change in the hormone receptor status.

There are a number of nutritional supplements available that can be extremely helpful in this process. A medical-grade multivitamin combined with calcium, magnesium and essential fatty acid (fish oil) is critical in diminishing the number and severity of symptoms that occur while one is stopping HRT and afterward. Regular exercise can make a huge difference in terms of the number and intensity of postmenopauseal or perimenopausal symptoms.

The use of black cohosh as well as soy (80–100 mg of isoflavones a day) may also help abate the symptoms of hot flashes. Be sure to avoid genetically modified soy; choose products labeled "Non-GMO." Soy has also been shown to be helpful in reducing the risk of heart disease; some studies have demonstrated improved bone density; and most recently, studies have shown its ability to decrease the response of insulin in the body, which is particularly important for those who are insulin resistant or diabetic.

Of concern for me is the fact that Wyeth, the manufacturer of Premarin and Prempro, petitioned the FDA in 2005 to restrict the availability of compounded "bio-identical" hormones.

I am grateful several, well-known celebrities have done a lot towards increasing awareness of bio-identical hormones. In 2009, Oprah Winfrey said menopause caught her "off guard" and that taking bioidentical hormones made a big improvement in how she felt. Oprah, when in her mid-fifties, wrote in *O, The Oprah Magazine* that she felt "out of kilter" and had "issues" for two years she suspected were hormonal. Upon a friend's recommendation, Winfrey went to a doctor who specialized in bioidentical hormone therapy. She noted after one day feeling like a veil was lifted. Oprah has done a lot to encourage women to "take charge of their health" and "start the conversation" about menopause and bioidentical hormones.

Suzanne Somers has done a lot to bring information out about bioidenitcal hormones as well. She has written several books and sings the praises of natural hormone therapy. *The Sexy Years,* by Suzanne Somers delivers helpful information about hormonal imbalances that menopause can bring and she has put bioidentical hormones on the map with media appearances on many shows from Home Shopping Network to the Larry King Show.

In particular, Somers draws from her friend, Dr. Diana Schwarzbein (author of The Schwarzbein Principle), an endocrinologist who uses natural, bioidentical hormones. Dr. Schwarzbein has drawn heavily from Dr. Lee's work over the years, and they even borrowed a slightly altered version of his Three Rules for Hormone Replacement for Somers' book, which you can find in the original on this website (http://www.johnleemd.com/thruforusbih.html).

There are a few things you should know about bioidentical hormones. One of them is that they are usually compounded. This means that they are formulated based on the precise specifications of a doctor who prescribes them. There are many medications that are compounded; bioidentical hormones are just one of the many. Some people say that there is an issue with compounded prescriptions and that they are not FDA approved.

The FDA doesn't approve any compounded products, for any condition, because those products can't be standardized. And, therein lays the beauty in the art of compounding. One size does not fill all when it comes to hormone therapy. I prescribe the lowest and most exact dose formula on symptoms to control those symptoms most effectively. Compounding can also be useful for patients who are allergic to an additive in an FDA-approved product. Because compounded products don't go through the FDA approval process, they don't bear the same warnings as other hormone therapy.

Just because the process is not approved does not mean the actual ingredients are not approved. They absolutely are. It is important that since compounding is a precise science that patients look for accredited compounding pharmacies listed on the web site of the Pharmaceutical Compounding Accreditation Board (PCAB). Since these accredited pharmacies can be hard to find, due to the stringent rules, patients should ask compounding pharmacies what types of quality assurance procedures are in place. Also you will need to ask for information on side effects and warnings because these may not be included when prescriptions are compounded.

It is not completely necessary you use compounded hormones. There are FDA-approved "bioidentical" drugs available. The biggest reason for using compounding is the customization of doses. Another reason to use compounding would be if someone has allergies to ingredients, or intolerances to doses, in commercially available products.

There is no reason to think bioidentical compounded products would have a different safety profile than the FDA-approved ones. You must be careful as some compounding pharmacies have gotten warning letters from the FDA for false and misleading claims about safety and other benefits.

Compounding pharmacies can formulate products into many forms including tablets, capsules, creams, gels, lozenges, suppositories and more. Compounding pharmacies create products from one or more active ingredients. The United States Pharmacopeia (USP) is the recognized national formulary and offers guidance for compounding. Ingredients, according to the USP, must meet quality standards; such as: pharmaceutical grade, reagent grade or even food grade. The active ingredients and inactive ingredients are specified by a licensed health care physician with a prescription.

The healthcare practitioner specifies ingredients and doses intended to meet the individual needs of their patients. For example these pharmacies can combine multiple bioidentical hormones of various strengths into one compounded medication. The prescriber will also specify the type of formulation to use. Flavoring can be added to formulations to make them more palatable, if desired.

The greatest success comes from an individualized approach. When warranted, we prescribe a precise dosage of bioidentical estrogen, testosterone or DHEA that is made up at a compounding pharmacy to alleviate individual symptoms and target specific issues to the individual. Each patient is then monitored carefully through regular follow-up. Treatment and adjustments should be based on symptoms and quality of life issues more than blood hormone levels. Lab tests (saliva or blood) are best to use to establish baselines, rule out serious disease/tumors, and to assess success of absorption into the system.

I get asked many times "How long will I need to be on Hormone therapy?"

The answer to this depends on how long you have symptoms or the body has issues consistent with hormone deficiencies. For some this is a few months, for others many years.

I also get asked about having periods after menopause. It is not necessary for a postmenopausal woman to have periods if she is using bioidentical hormones properly. When postmenopausal women use small doses of bioidentical hormones, they rarely, if ever, have periods. Nor do they have the risky endometrial buildup in the uterus which is what makes it important to have periods. Estrogen stimulates the buildup of uterine tissue, but there's no need to take that much estrogen to feel healthy and balanced. Since fat cells create estrogen, women who are heavy may not even need to use supplemental estrogen.

Dr. Lee's recommendation was always to use the lowest dose possible of any hormone supplementation. Usually this was 15 to 30 mg of progesterone daily, and the lowest dose of estrogen that would either clear up estrogen deficiency symptoms or show normal levels on a saliva hormone level test. This improves health and well-being, but doesn't put a postmenopausal woman back into the same hormonal milieu she had when she was menstruating every month.

When you take progesterone in a pill form, most of it goes directly to the liver, where up to 80 percent of it may be dumped, but not before creating a variety of byproducts (metabolites). Thus, it's necessary to take 100 mg of progesterone in pill form to get 20 mg into your cells. If your liver happens to be working less efficiently on a given day, and excretes less of the progesterone, it's easy to experience overdose side effects; such as, sleepiness and bloating. These side effects often have women running for more estrogen to wake themselves up again. What they really need to do is use progesterone cream, which is a much more efficient delivery method. If you put 20 mg on your skin, virtually all of that will be in your bloodstream within a matter of minutes.

Saliva Testing? What's that all about???

Saliva testing has become the most specific way to assess the hormone levels in your tissues. Blood tests show only fluctuating levels from minute to minute. A full assessment of multiple hormones can be tested. It is easy to do. Although some insurance does not pay for it; these tests can be more affordable than blood tests in some cases.

Saliva testing is a convenient, inexpensive, and above all, accurate means of testing steroid hormones. Scientific studies have shown a strong correlation between steroid hormone levels in saliva and the amount of hormone in the blood that is active or "bioavailable." Saliva is an ideal diagnostic medium to measure the bioavailable levels of steroid hormones active in the tissue. It is this fraction of total hormone that is free to enter the target tissues in the brain, uterus, skin, and breasts.

Saliva testing can be done anywhere, anytime. Testing that relies on blood drawn in the doctor's office makes it harder to obtain samples at specific times (such as in the early morning) or multiple times during the day. In addition, hormones in saliva are exceptionally stable and can be stored at room temperature for up to a week without affecting the accuracy of the result. This offers maximum flexibility in sample collection and shipment. Several of the steroid hormones can be tested in the saliva including, estradiol, estrone, estriol, progesterone, testosterone, DHEA-S, and cortisol.

When a woman experiences prolonged stress, pregnenolone (that comes from the precursor cholesterol), a hormone essential for both coping with stress and producing female hormones, is diverted from the normal hormone pathway. As a result, the production of female hormones is compromised. This condition can cause a multitude of symptoms including irritability, mood swings, headaches, sleeplessness, and weight gain.

Each person is different and the whole person and hormonal chemical make-up and balance are unique. The doctor must take into account all the different complexities of an individual's hormone make-up and balance and work with what the person has in their environment to maximize the hormonal balance.

The hormonal health of any woman depends upon the delicate dance of progesterone and estrogen. Estrogen is meant to be the predominant hormone in the first half of the menstrual cycle and progesterone the predominant one in the second half. However, for most women in the industrialized world this is not the case.

There are many causes of hormone imbalance, but at the base of the problem is something called Estrogen Dominance - which means there is too much estrogen and not enough progesterone present in the body. There are many symptoms that result from having low progesterone levels.

What follows is a look at some of the common ways in which medicine and industry have tampered with the natural balance of our hormones. Women have used these products blindly at the cost of our hormonal balance, overall health, and longevity. Some of these may be obvious to you, while some may come as a surprise. Either way the hormonal imbalances that result should not be taken lightly. They contribute to the rise in cancers, especially breast and ovarian cancers, heart disease, depression, pms and more.

The common causes of hormonal imbalance and estrogen dominance:

- Artificial hormone replacement therapy (The Pill and Prempro)
- Environmental poisons
- Non organic and estrogen pumped animal products
- Stress
- Cosmetics (chemicals in them that mimic estrogen in the body)

Progestins and progestogens (artificial progesterone) are highly toxic to the body, resulting in some of these known side effects:

- miscarriages
- migraines
- heart disease
- high blood pressure
- cancer
- depression

and, of course ... low progesterone, the true biologic levels.

These are some of the common ways that medicine has tampered with the natural balance of hormones, here are some the ways that industry has tampered with the same delicate hormonal balance.

Chemicals such as pesticides mimic the hormone estrogen. Fifty-one chemicals have now been identified as hormone disruptors. Approximately 2 billion tons of pesticides are used the annually the world over. In undeveloped countries, the use of pesticides is still largely unchecked and ... guess what? That is where we get a lot of our food supplies. It's plain to see why this is wreaking havoc on our bodies. It is this fact that has led many people to switch to an organic diet.

Other chemicals that cause the same challenges are DDT, dioxin and PCB's (polychlorinated biphenyls.) Dioxin is the by-product of the manufacture of chemicals using chlorine and includes:

- disinfectants
- dry cleaning fluids
- pesticides
- drugs
- plastics – polystyrene and cling wrap in particular

PCB's are used in:

- lubricants
- plastics
- paints
- varnishes
- inks

Commonly called petrochemicals, they contain high levels of xeno-estrogens. Xeno-estrogens basically mean they mimic estrogen in your body. They fill up all the estrogen receptor sites in your body; even the good estrogen can't get through to perform its role properly. This results in hormone imbalance. This is why many people have moved over to household cleaning products that don't contain these chemicals and are environment friendly. Non-organic animals that are slaughtered for our food chain are fed estrogenic steroids to fatten them up. These estrogens go straight into our blood stream causing a further rise in estrogen levels. Another study linked the increase of our current disease rates to eating a diet high in the fat and meat from these estrogen-fed animals. Again, it is this fact that has led many people to switch to an organic diet. Cosmetics may come as a surprise to you, but many cosmetics are made with petrochemicals, yes like you put in your car. It's not surprising then to realize that these 'moisturizers' are actually drying out your skin - actually causing more wrinkles!

Even more importantly they are further putting your hormones out of balance. Just to list a few aqueous cream, petroleum jelly, mineral oil, liquid paraffin, talc powders, parabens, and other estrogenic antioxidants

Again, this is why many people have moved over to moisturizers that don't contain these chemicals and are environment friendly.

As if all of the above where not enough, stress also plays a big part in reducing our levels of progesterone which results in … too much estrogen.

Here's how: Progesterone is the "mother of all hormones." It is the precursor and essential raw material out of which the body created

ALL THE OTHER HORMONES. As the precursor to all the other hormones in the body, the adrenal glands and adrenal hormones are no exception. If you encounter a mildly stressful situation your body draws on its progesterone to produce the hormones (adrenal corticosteroids) to counteract it. These are the hormones that protect against stress. BUT, if your body is in a constant or permanent state of stress it can't provide enough progesterone to be converted into anti-stress hormones and the result is adrenal exhaustion and no left over progesterone for other normal body functions. You can change your life!   You can restore balance. You can combat aging and ill health effects starting today. You must find someone knowledgeable about hormones and who will listen to you and your situation and find the right solution that fits only you.

Recommended online references:

http://www.womensinternational.com/
http://women.webmd.com/new
www.womentowomen.com
http://www.johnleemd.com
http://www.zrtlab.com/
http://www.lef.org
www.project-aware.org
http://www.pcab.info/

When it comes to hormones:

1. Don't assume
2. Understand your body
3. You are right to be reluctant about artificial HRT

Bioidentical hormones are already in our bodies. I have patients who need oxygen supplementation often tell me that they are afraid the will get "addicted" to oxygen if they start using a machine. This is so silly because we are all addicted to oxygen. We need it every second of every day. The same holds true with our hormones. We need them every second of every day and using natural hormones to supplement deficiencies cannot possibly cause you to become addicted to hormones. I am always careful to use the term supplementation, not replacement. You do not simply stop making sex steroid hormones after your ovaries fail and shrivel up. You still make hormones from your adrenal glands, the little guys on top of the kidneys, although, in much smaller amounts than if you have healthy active ovaries. Supplementing your body to bring you back in balance only makes sense in many circumstances.

The process of aging is accompanied by reduced levels of hormones that maintain our youth. With this decline, in both, men and women, heart disease, stroke, osteoporosis and chronic inflammatory and neurodegenerative disorders develop.

Men have problems with decreasing testosterone, as well. Mainstream medicine's ignorance regarding the need to maintain testosterone in the higher ranges is a significant cause of premature disability and death in aging men. Most people are in a state of denial about declining hormone levels. A 30 to 40 year old man is often shocked when his blood test results uncover strikingly low testosterone levels. I see it in my practice all the time, especially, if they are overweight.

HDL is the "good cholesterol" and protects against atherosclerosis and heart disease. Testosterone plays a critical role in helping HDL to remove the built-up bad cholesterol away from the arterial wall.

Testosterone is required for optimal transport of excess cholesterol from our tissues and blood vessels to our liver for processing and disposal. In the testosterone-deficient state, reverse cholesterol transport is compromised, and excess cholesterol cannot be removed from the arterial wall.

One of the biggest barriers for testosterone supplementation is the fear of prostate cancer. However, this need not be a fear because hundreds of clinical trials have shown that low testosterone is more of a risk factor than high testosterone levels and men with low testosterone levels have an increased percentage of prostate cancer-positive biopsies. It has been shown that as free testosterone levels decline in aging men, their PSA levels sharply increase. Even though it is clear that testosterone does not cause prostate cancer, I still advise avoidance of testosterone until the disease is cured in a male with active untreated diagnosed prostate cancer.

Another problem with hormonal imbalance is that excess abdominal fat is a major culprit in many men with high estradiol levels. Excess body fat, particularly in the abdominal region is a major factor in imbalanced estrogen metabolism. Abdominal obesity increases aromatase activity, which increases estradiol, which in excess causes more abdominal fat. A negative feedback loop is established and health suffers as a result. Reducing abdominal fat will mitigate excessive estradiol levels. Zinc is very helpful in the process of reversing this loop. Wheat germ is an excellent, high-potency vegetarian source of zinc.

Zinc also functions as an aromatase inhibitor in many men. Although red meats are a primary source of zinc, non-meat sources such as wheat germ or roasted pumpkin and squash seeds compare quite favorably with the levels found in animal protein sources. For estradiol balance, zinc can be supplemented at 80mg per day. DIM (di-indolmethane) is derived from the phytochemical IC3 (Indole-3-Carbinol). DIM works by converting estradiol into a less potent, and less harmful, form of estrogen called estriol. Although both DIM and IC3 can be found in nutrient supplement forms, IC3 is also found naturally in cruciferous vegetables such as cabbage, broccoli and kale. In supplement form, DIM is more easily absorbed into the body.

In males, the main biologically active estrogen is estradiol. The primary source of estradiol in men is from the conversion (aromatization) of testosterone. As men age, the production of androgens from the adrenals and gonads is decreased. The aromatization of testosterone to estradiol is often maintained, but due to a variety of factors, more testosterone is aromatized in fatty tissues, causing a further imbalance of the ratio of testosterone to estrogen, i.e. too much estradiol and not enough testosterone. The result is a deficiency of beneficial testosterone and an excess amount of estradiol.

As men age, the amount of testosterone produced in the testes diminishes greatly. Yet estradiol levels remain persistently high. The reason for this is increasing aromatase activity along with age-associated fat mass, especially in the belly.

Estradiol levels correlate significantly to body fat mass and more specifically to subcutaneous abdominal fat. The epidemic of abdominal obesity observed in aging men is associated with a constellation of degenerative disorders, including heart disease, diabetes, and cancer.

Subcutaneous abdominal fat acts as a secretory gland, often producing and emitting excessive levels of estradiol into an aging man's blood. One's waist circumference is a highly accurate prognostic measurement of future disease risk. Excess estradiol secretion is at least one of the deadly mechanisms associated with the difficult-to-resolve problem of having too much abdominal fat. Symptoms of excess estrogen in aging men include the development of breasts, having too much abdominal weight, feeling tired, suffering loss of muscle mass, and having emotional disturbances. Many of these symptoms correspond to testosterone deficiency as well.

Both men and women need estrogen to maintain bone density, cognitive function, and even to maintain the inner lining of the arterial wall (the endothelium). Both men and women with declining hormone levels are at increased risk of osteoporosis, a condition that means your bones are weak, and you're more likely to break a bone. Since there are no symptoms, you might not know your bones are getting weaker until you break a bone. A broken bone can cause disability, pain, or loss of independence.

With the decline of the female hormone estrogen at menopause, usually around age 50, bone breakdown markedly increases. For several years, women lose bone two to four times faster than they did before menopause. The rate usually slows down again, but some women may continue to lose bone rapidly. By age 65, some women have lost half their skeletal mass.

The FDA has approved several kinds of devices that use various methods to estimate bone density. A newer technique for evaluating bone strength is ultrasound and the FDA has approved several instruments for this purpose. The devices for ultrasound measurement are cheaper and easier to use. This makes them available in more locations and allows evaluation for osteoporosis in many more subjects. Another new test provides an indicator of bone breakdown. In 1995, the FDA approved a simple, noninvasive biochemical test that detects in a urine sample a specific component of bone breakdown, called NTx.

Calcium and vitamin D supplements are an integral part of all treatments for osteoporosis. Healthy diet and exercise are important not only for treatment, but also for prevention. A lifelong habit of weight-bearing exercise, such as walking or biking, also helps build and maintain strong bone. The greatest benefit for older people is that physical fitness reduces the risk of fracture. Better balance, muscle strength, and agility make falls less likely. People who don't consume dairy foods can meet their calcium needs with foods that are fortified with calcium, such as orange juice, or with calcium supplements. Other good sources of calcium are dark-green leafy vegetables like kale and turnip greens, tofu (if made with calcium), canned fish (eaten with bones), and fortified cereal products. Women over the age of 50 should have at least 1200 mg/ day and women form 19-50 should have about 1000 mg.

Chapter 5

"Taming the Master"
Thyroid Balance and Adequate Iodine

The thyroid gland sits in your mid neck, is shaped like a butterfly, and consists of two lobes that lie on each side of the trachea (windpipe) located just below the Adam's apple. It's one of the largest endocrine glands in the body and is also one of the most amazing and sensitive. This unique mass of specialized tissue produces the thyroid hormones thyroxine (T4) and triiodothyronine (T3), the primary regulators of human metabolism. The numbers 4 & 3 after the "T" designate the number of iodine atoms they each contain. Both hormones are derived from the amino acid tyrosine. Thyroid hormones accelerate cellular reactions and increase oxidative metabolism, by stimulating enzymes that control active transport pumps, demand for cellular oxygen increases, and as ATP production goes up and heat is produced. This creates a thermoregulatory effect, which increases body temperature.

Basal metabolic rate (BMR) is directly influenced by thyroid hormone biochemistry. Thyroid hormones can target, influence and alter the metabolism of virtually every cell in the body. They affect mood, bodyweight, stamina and even fertility. Thyroid hormones stimulate protein synthesis and increase the rate at which triglycerides are broken down (lipolysis) affecting the appearance of the bodies muscle physique and help preserve muscle and reduce body fat. When used incorrectly and/or excessively, they are highly catabolic to muscle or have the opposite effect. This is why it is not recommended to use thyroid supplementation just for aesthetics, it is too difficult to over use and have the reverse of what you want and why it is important to monitor levels in the blood to achieve desired results.

Synthetic forms of pure thyroxine (Synthroid, Levothroid, Levoxyl) rate high on the list of drugs most frequently prescribed by physicians. They can stimulate appetite, speed metabolic rate and help people lose weight, but if abused or used incorrectly, they can also cause serious heart problems, muscle weakness and muscle wasting. Alternatives to T4 alone include synthetic T3 (Cytomel) and desiccated animal gland extracts that contain both T4 & T3 (Armour, Naturthroid, Westroid). All forms may be useful depending on the individual and thyroid condition. The solution is to determine the best dose, form and combination.

The thyroid secretes about ten times as much T4 as T3; however, T3 is roughly 2-3 times more potent. Thyroxine is converted into the more active triiodothyronine with the selenium dependent enzyme 5'-deiodinase. Thus, some thyroid disorders are simply a consequence of consuming a diet that lacks sufficient selenium. T3 and T4 are lipid-soluble and combine with special transport proteins upon release into the serum, called thyroxine-binding globulins (TBG). Less than 1% of thyroid hormones travel unattached in their free state.

During growth, thyroid hormones provide an anabolic influence on protein metabolism. This is due to their influence on insulin secretion. T4 and insulin also connect in the liver, where they mutually affect IGF activity. IGF (Insulin Growth Factors) are powerful muscle building control agents. In the absence of adequate levels of thyroid hormones, human growth hormone (hGH) also loses its growth-promoting action and is not secreted normally.

Thyroid problems are incredibly common in North America, especially among women. As a RULE, when all else fails and you can't figure out what's wrong, suspect low thyroid and get it tested ASAP. Many experts believe this epidemic is caused by excess chemicals in our food, air and water. All of these stress the immune system leading to a high incidence of autoimmune illness. Common symptoms of low thyroid include unusual fatigue, susceptibility to feeling cold, trouble with weight management, prominent bags under eyes, muscle and joint aches and pains, problems with digestion, mental sluggishness, dry skin, depression, migraines and waking up feeling tired. Instead of feeling refreshed after a morning workout, you might feel like going back to bed (even though it's only 10am). Or, after work instead of heading to the gym, you head straight home because you feel completely drained. Athletes with low thyroid do not perform well when the ambient temperature drops below 50° F. The synovial fluid in the joints also tends to "thicken", thus reducing joint motility and increasing risk of injury.

Women typically under consume protein, especially low-fat, non-denatured animal protein, which provides a strong source of the essential amino acid phenylalanine. Tyrosine is known as the "anti-stress" amino, and is greatly depleted after hard workouts and exhausting sport competition. Thyroid hormones depend on ample pools of tyrosine, which is dependent on phenylalanine intake. Fortunately, tyrosine can be taken directly in supplement form.

Women are prone to anemia or iron deficiency through menstrual cycles which can exacerbate thyroid problems because iron influences thyroid function. Anemia induced through iron deficiency has been shown to significantly reduce circulating levels of T4-5'deiodinase, resulting in suppression of the conversion of T4 to T3 thereby resulting in low plasma T4 levels. After 12 weeks of iron supplementation, and iron deficiency correction, both T4 levels and the ability of the body to thermoregulate body temperature following exposure to cold improves.

The thyroid gland is the main metabolic regulator of our bodies. To convert thyroxine (T4) the inactive form to triiodthyronine (T3) the active form requires the removal of an iodine molecule from T4 and adequate stores of iodine are needed to then make more T4. This process also requires the mineral selenium, vitamin A, vitamin E, zinc and iron and without them can imitate iodine deficiency.

Some symptoms of iodine deficiency are: cognitive impairment, fibrocystic breast disease, goiter, hyperthyroidism, hypothyroidism, and miscarriages.

How many times have I heard, "My doctor tested my thyroid and it was fine."? The problem is many people recognize that the thyroid regulates metabolism, but are not educated or empowered enough to go one step further. To this day, I do not understand why so many doctors think that TSH (thyroid stimulating hormone) blood tests are the only way to diagnose thyroid problems. When I was an X-ray tech, we were taught that "one view was no view". This meant that when we did an X-ray of a chest, if you only did a front to back view this was not enough information. You had to do a side view, as well. We called this a 2-view chest. You can't see through the tissues the other way and the same was with extremities like arms and legs. You might miss a fracture if you didn't get the other views or angles. Well lab testing is the same way. One test is NO test! You have to have the rest of the information to make a diagnosis, to see the whole picture. You have to understand what the tests mean too. You must also recognize that "normal" values are a bell curve or an average of patients tested who are "normal". Does that mean if you are one point outside the range that suddenly you are "abnormal"? This is crazy to think such an arbitrary cut off can make you normal or abnormal or rule in or out disease.

Many endocrinologists (specialists who deal with hormonal issues) are known for being "numbers" people. They manage by the numbers, and not by the symptoms. This method can often create the "you're in the normal range, so you're fine" response from doctors when many of us complain we still don't feel well. Keep in mind, if you have easily diagnosed hypothyroidism, it may take some serious looking to find an endocrinologist who believes in finding an optimal TSH for you.

Diagnosing thyroid disease is a process that can incorporate numerous factors, including clinical evaluation, blood tests, imaging tests, biopsies and other tests. Many thyroid diseases exist beyond just a "hypofunctioning" gland. These include: hypothyroidism, Hashimoto's Disease, Hyperthyroidism: Graves' Disease, goiter (enlarged gland) and nodules (lumpy gland).

Here is a list of different blood tests used to diagnose thyroid issues.

- Thyroid Stimulating Hormone (TSH) Test
- Total T4(Thyroxine)
- Free T4(Thyroxine)

- Total T3(Triiodothyronine)
- Free T3 (Triiodothyronine)
- Thyroglobulin(Thyroid Binding Globulin/TBG)
- T3 Resin Uptake(T3RU)
- Reverse T3
- Thyroid Peroxidase Antibodies (TPOAb)(Antithyroid Peroxidase Antibodies)
- Antithyroid Microsomal Antibodies(Antimicrosomal Antibodies)
- Thyroglobulin Antibodies(Antithyroglobulin Antibodies)
- Thyroid Receptor Antibodies(TRAb)
- Thyroid-Stimulating Immunoglobulins(TSI)

TSH blood Test - The most common thyroid test is the blood test that measures the amount of thyroid-stimulating hormone (TSH) in your bloodstream. Here's where it gets tricky! If the TSH is elevated or high, we think hypothyroidism or low function. If the TSH is low, then this is usually evidence of hyperthyroidism. This may seem a little backwards, but TSH is a hormone from that brain that has a "feedback effect" on the thyroid gland. So, when the TSH is elevated you may have a low thyroid function. When it is low, you may have an overly functioning thyroid.

Free T4 / Free Thyroxine - Free T4 measures the free, unbound thyroxine levels in your bloodstream. Free T4 is typically elevated in hyperthyroidism and lowered in hypothyroidism. Free or unbound T4 levels represent the level of hormone available for uptake and use by cells. Bound levels represent a circulating hormone that may not all be immediately available, because it is affected by other drugs, illness, and physical changes such as pregnancy. Because the free levels of T4 represent immediately available hormone, free T4 is thought to better reflect the patient's available hormonal status than total T4.

Total T4/Total Thyroxine - This test measures the total amount of circulating thyroxine in your blood. Thyroxine, a hormone produced by the thyroid, is also known as T4. A high value can indicate hyperthyroidism; a low value can indicate hypothyroidism. Total T4 levels can be elevated due to pregnancy and other high estrogen states, including use of estrogen replacement or birth control pills.

Total T3/Total Triiodothyronine - Triiodothyronine is the active thyroid hormone and is also known as T3. Total T3 is typically elevated in hyperthyroidism and lowered in hypothyroidism.

Free T3 / Free Triiodothyronine - Free T3 measures the free, unbound levels of triiodothyronine in your bloodstream. Free T3 is considered more accurate than Total T3. Free T3 is typically elevated in hyperthyroidism and lowered in hypothyroidism.

T3 Resin Uptake (T3RU) – Just one more piece of the puzzle. Not used a lot but when done with a T3 and T4, the T3 resin uptake (T3RU) test is sometimes referred to as the T7 test. This test measures the amount of unsaturated binding sites on the transport (binding) hormones. The T3RU test measures the level of proteins that carry thyroid hormone in the blood. Elevated T3RU is more commonly seen with hyperthyroidism. Keep in mind, certain medications like steroids, heparin, phenytoin, aspirin, and Coumadin can increase T3RU values and male androgen replacement, illness and kidney disease can increase thyroxin binding globulin (TBG) levels. There are drugs that can decrease T3RU values like antithyroid medications, birth control pills, clofibrate, estrogen, and thiazides. Pregnancy can also decrease T3RU levels.

Thyroglobulin/Tg - Thyroglobulin (Tg) levels are low or undetectable with normal thyroid function but can by elevated in thyroiditis, Graves' disease, or thyroid cancer. Monitoring of Tg levels is frequently used as a tumor marker to evaluate the effectiveness of treatment for thyroid cancer and to monitor for thyroid cancer recurrence.

Reverse T3 - When the body is under stress, instead of converting T4 into T3 - the active form of thyroid hormone - the body conserves energy by making what is known as Reverse T3 (RT3), an inactive form of the T3 hormone. The value of RT3 tests in diagnosis is controversial, as some practitioners believe that the body continues to manufacture RT3 instead of active T3, causing various symptoms that are identified as Wilson's syndrome or symptomatic low function thyroid issues.

Thyroid Peroxidase (TPO) Antibodies (TPOAb) / Antithyroid Peroxidase Antibodies - Thyroid Peroxidase (TPO) antibodies, are also known as Antithyroid Peroxidase Antibodies. (In the past, these antibodies were referred to as Antithyroid Microsomal Antibodies or Antimicrosomal Antibodies). These antibodies work against thyroid peroxidase, an enzyme that plays a part in the T4-to-T3 conversion and synthesis process. TPO antibodies can be evidence of tissue destruction, such as Hashimoto's disease, less commonly, in other forms of thyroiditis such as post-partum thyroiditis. It's estimated that TPO antibodies are detectable in approximately 95 percent of patients with Hashimoto's thyroiditis and 50 to 85 percent of Graves' disease patients. The concentrations of antibodies found in patients with Graves' disease are usually lower than in patients with Hashimoto's disease.

Thyroglobulin Antibodies / Antithyroglobulin Antibodies - Testing for thyroglobulin antibodies (also called antithyroglobulin antibodies) is common. If you have already been diagnosed with Graves' disease, having high levels of thyroglobulin antibodies means that you are more likely to eventually become hypothyroid. Thyroglobulin antibodies are positive in about 60 percent of Hashimoto's patients and 30 percent of Graves' patients.

Thyroid-Stimulating Immunoglobulins (TSI) / TSH Stimulating Antibodies (TSAb) - TSH receptor antibodies (TRAb) are seen in most patients with a history of, or who currently have, Graves' disease. Testing is usually done for a specific type of stimulating TRAb that goes by several different names, including: Thyroid-Stimulating Immunoglobulins (TSI) and TSH stimulating antibodies (TSAb). Thyroid-stimulating immunoglobulins (TSI) can be detected in the majority - some estimates say as many as 75 to 90 percent - of Graves' disease patients. The higher the levels, the more active the Graves' disease is thought to be. (The absence of these antibodies does not, however, rule out Graves' disease.) Less commonly, some people with Hashimoto's disease also have these antibodies, and this can cause periodic short term episodes of hyperthyroidism. When monitoring TSI, elevated levels may help predict relapse of Graves' disease, and lowered TSI levels may indicate that Graves' disease treatment is working.

TRH test- If hypothyroidism symptoms are present, but TSH tests are normal the physician measures the patient's TSH level (a simple blood test), gives an injection of TRH, then draws blood 25 minutes later and remeasures the TSH. If the first TSH level is normal and the second TSH level is high (greater than 10) the patient's thyroid is underactive. A TSH reading of 15 is suspicious, while 20 strongly points to hypothyroidism. If you have three or more typical symptoms of underactive thyroid but have tested 'normal' in standard tests, 35-40% actually have underactive thyroids based on the TRH test."

Some of the tests that are used to diagnose thyroid disease are:

Nuclear Scan / Radioactive Iodine Uptake (RAI-U) - A radioactive iodine uptake (RAI-U) test can help tell whether a person has Graves' disease, toxic multinodular goiter, or thyroiditis. In this test, a small dose of radioactive iodine 123 (radiotracer) is given in pill form. Several hours later, the amount of iodine accumulates in the thyroid and gives off energy in the form of gamma rays. This energy is detected by a device called gamma camera or a PET scanner. A computer then produces special pictures that give details of the structure and function of the thyroid gland.

Intake of high amounts of iodine in your diet can interfere with the test results including medications or supplements that contain iodine, such as multivitamins, kelp, and seaweed. Also, keep in mind, if you've had medical tests that used iodine contrast dyes, this may skew your RAI-U results for weeks or months and make the test results less accurate. An overactive thyroid, usually, takes up higher amounts of iodine than normal. A thyroid that takes up iodine is considered "hot," or overactive, as opposed to a "cold" or underactive thyroid. In Graves' disease, RAI-U is elevated, and the entire gland becomes hot. In Hashimoto's thyroiditis, the uptake is usually low with patchy hot spots in the gland. RAI-U can show when thyroid nodules are hot. If you are hyperthyroid due to a hot nodule, and not Graves' disease, the nodule will show up as hot, and the rest of your thyroid will be cold. Hot nodules may overproduce thyroid hormone but they are rarely cancerous. RAI-U can also show which thyroid nodules are cold - not taking up iodine - and an estimated 10 to 20 percent of cold nodules are cancerous.

CT Scan - A CT scan, known as computed tomography or "cat scan," is a specialized type of 3-D x-ray that is sometimes used to evaluate the thyroid. A CT scan can't detect smaller nodules, but may help detect and diagnose a goiter, or larger thyroid nodules.

MRI / Magnetic Resonance Imaging - MRI is done when the size and shape of the thyroid needs to be evaluated. MRI can't tell how the thyroid is functioning (i.e., it can't diagnose hyperthyroidism or hypothyroidism), but it can detect enlargement. It is sometimes preferable to x-rays or CT scans because it doesn't require any injection of contrast dye, and doesn't require radiation.

Thyroid Ultrasound - Ultrasound of the thyroid is done to evaluate nodules, lumps and enlargement of your gland. Ultrasound can tell whether a nodule is a fluid-filled cyst or a mass of solid tissue. It cannot determine if a nodule or lump is malignant. Because the thyroid typically enlarges in Graves' disease, and the gland typically reduces when responding to antithyroid drug treatment, some practitioners use ultrasound to monitor the success of antithyroid treatment.

To completely evaluate your thyroid function, your doctor should do the following:

Feel your thyroid gland for lumps, nodules, enlargement or "thrills" rushing of blood through it

Listen to your thyroid using a stethoscope for bruits or sounds of increased blood flow in the thyroid

Test your reflexes at the knee and ankle with a hammer to see if your reflexes are over or underactive. Hyper-responsive reflexes can be a sign of hyperthyroidism, and slow reflexes may point to hypothyroidism.

Check your heart rate, rhythm, and blood pressure. A slow heart rate (bradycardia) may point to hypothyroidism. A high heart rate (tachycardia), high blood pressure, or rhythm irregularites may point to hyperthyroidism.

Measure your weight. Rapid weight gain, without a change to diet or exercise can be a sign of hypothyroidism. Rapid weight loss may point to hyperthyroidism.

Measure body temperature. Low body temperature might be a possible sign of an underactive thyroid.

Examine your face, looking for loss of hair in the outer edge of the eyebrows -- a symptom of hypothyroidism -- as well as puffiness or swelling in the eyelids or face, another common hypothyroidism symptom. The eyes are often affected in thyroid patients. Common clinical symptoms include: bulging or protrusion of the eyes; a stare in the eyes; retraction of upper eyelids; a wide-eyed look; infrequent blinking; and "lid lag" -- when the upper eyelid doesn't smoothly follow downward movements of the eyes when you look down. Dull facial expression, hoarseness, or swelling in the face, hands or feet can be a sign of thyroid disorder.

Observe the general quantity and quality of your hair as hair loss is seen in both overactive and underactive thyroid. Coarse, brittle, or straw-like hair can point to hypothyroidism. Thinning, finer hair may point to hyperthyroidism.

Examine your skin as thyroid disease, especially hyperthyroidism, can show up in a variety of skin-related symptoms that include yellowish, jaundiced cast to the skin; unusually smooth, young-looking skin; hives; lesions or patches of rough skin on the shins (known as pretibial myxedema or Graves' dermopathy); or blister-like bumps of the forehead and face (known as milaria bumps).

Examine your nails and hands looking for hyperthyroidism related clinical signs in your nails and hands, including: Onycholysis or separation of the nail from the underlying nail bed, also called Plummer's nails, swollen fingertips or acropachy.

Review Other Clinical Signs of hyperthyroidism, including: tremors, shaky hands, Hyperkinetic movements like table drumming, tapping feet, jerky movements. Tests that may not be considered thyroid evaluations like bone density (DEXA scan or x-ray) as low bone density may be helpful to evaluate thyroid issues.

If a problem is found, your doctor may want to do a biopsy of the thyroid gland lesion. A needle biopsy, also known as fine needle aspiration (FNA) is used to help evaluate lumps or cold nodules. In a needle biopsy, a thin needle is inserted directly into the lump, some cells are withdrawn and they are evaluated for cancer. Often the doctors use ultrasound while conducting a biopsy in order to ensure the needle goes into the right position. Cancer can be definitively diagnosed about 75 percent of the time from FNA. Evaluation of biopsy results can also show cells indicative of Hashimoto's thyroiditis.

Some less mainstream tests that may be used are:

1. Iodine Patch Tests – paint a 1 inch square on your inner arm of iodine and watch to see how long it takes to absorb. Less than 1 hour and you may have an iodine deficiency.

2. Saliva Testing – for hormones and blood spot

3. Urinary Testing – for idodine

4. Basal Body Temperature Testing - Before going to bed at night - place a basal thermometer on your bedside table. As soon as you wake-up, place the thermometer in the centre of your armpit and then lay still for about 10 minutes. Record your body temperature and repeat this procedure for 3 consecutive days. Women should do this test during the first few days after menstruation begins. Add the three temperatures together and divide by 3. This figure represents your average basal metabolic temperature, which is reflective of thyroid hormone output. A normal temperature is approximately 37° C (98° F). Although "normal" does vary from person to person, a reading 1° or more below this range could indicate a problem with your thyroid.

Some patients need to be highly involved in their thyroid diagnosis and care. Self-tests and the ability to order your own tests can be a critical tool for an empowered patient.

Some things you can do at home to aid in detecting thyroid problems are:
Self neck, thyroid checks. To do this, hold a mirror up so you can see your thyroid area - the neck, just below the Adam's apple and above the collarbone. Tip your head back and keeping an eye on this thyroid area, take a drink of water and swallow. As you swallow, look at your neck. Watch carefully for any bulges,

enlargement, protrusions, or unusual appearances in this area. Repeat this process several times. If you see any bulges, protrusions, lumps or anything that appears unusual, see your doctor right away.

Fingerstick home blood tests through several different companies including Biosafe, ZRT, Diagnostechs and HealthCheckUSA.com that may include Anti-Thyroid Antibodies (Thyroglobulin Antibodies and Thyroid Peroxidase Antibodies), Thyroid panels that include T3 Uptake, T4 Total, T7, TSH, Free T3, Free T4, TSI (Thyroid Stimulating Immunoglobulin), and antimicrosomal antibodies. You order a test kit, which is sent to your home. You perform a simple fingerstick to collect a small drop of blood and then mail the test kit back to the company. You typically receive results within a week.

Being informed and knowledgeable about thyroid disease signs, symptoms, and risks can be an important part of getting properly diagnosed. Diagnosis of various thyroid disease and conditions involves clinical examination, blood tests, and in some cases, imaging tests and/or biopsy.

So, if you have low functioning thyroid issues, what are your treatment options? Synthroid, Levoxyl, Levothyroid, Euthyrox, Eltroxin are all brand names for the thyroid drug levothyroxine sodium, which is a synthetic version of the thyroid hormone T4. Remember that T4 is the inactive form of thyroid hormone and must be converted to T3. These are the drugs prescribed for thyroid hormone replacement for most patients. If you have hypothyroidism and are taking one of these conventional thyroid replacement drugs, your blood tests show a "normal" TSH, and, yet, you still don't feel well, there may be a need for the addition of T3 or active form of thyroid hormone.

If you have the inability to adequately convert T4 to the T3 needed by the body, you may still have a normal TSH, but present many hypothyroid symptoms. Serum hormone studies typically show marginally low T3 and T4 levels, usually within the "normal" range, and TSH is rarely elevated out of the "normal range." At the same time, cholesterol is often elevated, and basal temperature is likely to be 97 degrees F or less. Patients with hypometabolism problems often respond well to T3 or T4/T3 treatments.

Some scientists believe this may be the underlying cause of fibromylagia symptoms. Researchers have found higher incidence of thyroid disease among fibromylagia patients. And the researchers are also finding these patients need the additional thyroid hormone T3 to resolve symptoms.

T3 is available on its own, as a brand name drug known as Cytomel, or can be included with T4 in the naturally derived thyroid drug Armour Thyroid, or the synthetic version of Armour, which is known as Thyrolar.

Tyrosine, EFAs, Whey Protein Isolate, Selenium, Iron, Thyroid Glandular (desiccated thyroid with active ingredients removed), Glutamine & Lipoic Acid are specific to the problem at hand. Protein shakes are advised both before and after exercise. This is also a good time to add 1-2 tsp. of The Sport Oil, which helps ensure a reliable source of alpha-linolenic acid (omega-3). EFAs and whey protein isolate make a perfect pair to support nourishment of the entire endocrine gland system.

It is not recommended you use thyroid replacement for weight loss alone. You may make some issues worse or create new issues. If you have symptoms of low thyroid function and are overweight, than to not use some form of thyroid support will leave you spinning your wheels.

You owe it to yourself to understand your thyroid. Here are a few questions you may want to ask yourself.

Do you find that no matter how much you sleep, you're always waking up exhausted?

Do you feel like you have cobwebs in your head or constant brain fog?

Do you feel like even though you watch your diet, cut out junk food and exercise, the scale won't budge or you even gain weight?

Do you lose hair or does it feel thinner? Do you see it when you clean out the shower drain?

Do you battle depression or anxiety?

After childbirth, did you fail to lose "baby weight"?

Do you have ice-cold hands or feet?

Do you have dry skin?

Do you have insomnia or a poor sleep quality?

Do you have tingling in hands and feet?

Do you have muscle pain?

Do you have edema (swelling in ankles, legs or hands)?

Do you have elevated cholesterol?

All the symptoms above can be caused by an under-active thyroid or hypothyroidism. It can start as early as our middle 20s, getting progressively worse as we age.

Many people think thyroid when they think tired. So, they go to their doctor and try to talk about it. Your doctor humors you by giving you a thyroid blood test. Of course, when it comes back, you'll be told your thyroid is normal. You'll then be told it's "all in your head" and be given a prescription for anti-depressants. When a lab test is done, any result within a wide range is deemed normal. Your thyroid could be functioning at 30% of peak efficiency, even though it is within that "normal" range.

Taking an anti-depressant won't do a thing for your symptoms or your condition. Certainly, it will make the big drug companies very happy in having yet another long term customer hooked on their products.

You can increase your thyroid function with a simple but vital supplement: Iodine. Just how important is iodine?

Iodine is essential to a proper functioning thyroid. As we grow older, our thyroid starts slowing down. It just can't metabolize the iodine it needs as efficiently, and that means the hormone produced (also known as thyroid) goes down as well. There are many reasons why we might be iodine deficient, including: inadequate dietary intake and exposure to substances that displace iodine. Dietary intake is limited by the fact that iodine is a mineral and is not abundant in the food we eat. It can be found in very small quantities in seawater and soils close by but the further you get from the ocean the more limited the resource. Iodine exists naturally in most soils, and is taken up by plants, which in turn are eaten by humans and animals. Iodine is also fairly easily displaced from your body by toxins called toxic halides which include fluoride, bromine and chloride.

Fluoride is by far the worst culprit. Found in toothpaste and in your water supply, every time you take a shower, brush your teeth or drink from the tap, your body gets a little exposure to fluoride leeching out good iodine.

Fluoride may have its place to prevent tooth decay, but clearly it affects our iodine stores. Due to these factors, 96% of all people tested are iodine deficient. The World Health Organization also concurs, estimating that 72% of the world's population is being affected by iodine deficiency. Over the last 30 years iodine levels have dropped 50% in the U.S.A. alone.

The bottom line is that if there is not enough iodine in the thyroid gland, then it is impossible to have sufficient thyroid hormone of any type. The result is an under active thyroid or hypothyroidism.

Here's where it gets a little tricky. There are two types of iodine necessary for optimal nutrition and thyroid function: Iodine and iodide. The iodine supplements you normally find are made from kelp or seaweed lacking in iodide. Plus, the iodine supplements you'll see on the retail shelves are about 100 times weaker than they need to be. Iodine is present and used in every single cell in your body, including salivary glands, cerebrospinal fluid and the brain, gastric mucosa, choroid plexus (part of the brain), breasts, ovaries, and eye ciliary bodies.

Most studies recommend a full 5 mg of Iodine combined with a balanced amount of 7.5 mg of Iodide for the optimal formulation for peak bio-availability along with selenium which enhances conversion of the inactive thyroid hormone T4 into the active thyroid hormone T3.

If you are currently taking a thyroid hormone like Synthroid, Levothroid, Levoxyl or Armour, taking the iodine tablets will actually reduce the amount of your prescription dosage needed or may even eliminate it altogether.

If you are taking these prescription medications, please make sure you consult with your physician and take regular thyroid blood level tests.

My favorite form of iodine, Iodoral, can be purchased on line at Amazon.com, Naturamart.com and Life extension.com or at health food stores.

Iodoral is a tablet containing iodine and iodide as the potassium salt. To prevent gastric irritation, the iodine/iodide preparation is absorbed into a colloidal silica excipient. To eliminate the unpleasant taste of iodine, which is one of the major problems with liquid iodine supplement like Lugol's solution, the tablets are coated with a thin film of pharmaceutical glaze.

For adults, the recommended daily allowance is 150 micrograms, if you do not have symptoms of underactive thyroid function. Most of the human body's stores of iodine are located in the thyroid gland which requires it for the synthesis of thyroid hormones.

Sometimes, patients tell me they can't take iodine because they are allergic. Allergic reactions to iodine, usually, stem from iodine--based contrast dyes injected to sharpen pictures in medical imaging studies, such as x-rays and CT scans. These reactions, typically, are mild and involve nausea, vomiting, itching, flushing and hives. But in some cases, reactions can be quite severe (anaphylaxis) with swelling of the throat, difficulty breathing, profound low blood pressure, convulsions, and cardiac arrest. If you've experienced a severe reaction as a result of the dye used for an imaging study, make sure your physician and the radiologist supervising any future x-rays or scans are fully aware of your history.

A reaction to an iodine-based dye is not the same thing as an allergy to iodine because it generally doesn't stem from the same type of immune-system response as a true allergy. Having a reaction to an iodine-based contrast dye is also not the same as an allergy to seafood, which may be rich in iodine. If you're reacting to shellfish, the iodine it contains is unlikely to be responsible. It is more likely due to distinctive allergens found in these foods.

Most people who are allergic to shellfish react to certain proteins these foods contain, not to iodine. You can be allergic to all types of shellfish or only to one certain kind like mollusks (which include clams and oysters) or crustaceans (that include crabs and shrimp). Each of these two general types of shellfish contains different proteins. There is a small chance (about three percent) that if you're allergic to seafood, you'll have a reaction to contrast dye, but this is no more likely to happen than it is among people with other types of food allergies.

In general, if you reacted to an iodine-based contrast dye, you should be able to safely eat seafood and other foods high in iodine. If your reaction was to shellfish of some type, you are probably allergic to something other than iodine. And don't worry about your thyroid.

Your body will get the trace amounts of iodine needed to make thyroid hormone from your diet.

So, now that you know you need iodine for conversion of inactive to the active form of thyroid, you need to understand the traditional approach is to use synthetic hormones like Synthroid / Levoxyl / Levothroid (levothyroxine). These products only contain T4 hormone; they have no T3.

The common argument the physicians give is that the synthetic provides steady hormone levels. What the doctors tend to overlook is that the vast majority of people can not convert the T4 to the active form of thyroid which is T3. This is easy to confirm by measuring the free hormone levels.

When one has low T3 levels, which are typical with synthetic hormone use, the brain does not work properly. It is important to use a preparation with T3 because T3 does 90% of the work of the thyroid in the body. So, one should use a combination of T4 and T3 which compensates for the inability to convert T4 to T3. Armour thyroid is desiccated thyroid and has both T3 and T4.

Another issue with Armour is it is most effective when dosed twice a day. The most common starting dose for patients with hypothyroidism is 90 mg which is cut in half and taken after breakfast and the other half after dinner. Taking it after meals also helps to reduce volatility of the blood-level of T3. The TSH, Free T3 and Free T4 are then repeated in one month and the dose is adjusted.

Taking the Armour thyroid twice a day overcomes traditional medicine's major objection and resistance to using natural thyroid preparations – its variability in its blood-levels. Most doctors using Armour thyroid are not aware that Armour thyroid should be used twice daily and NOT once a day. The major reason is the T3 component has such a short half life and needs to be taken twice daily to achieve consistent blood levels. The best way to adjust the thyroid hormone is to increase the dosage until the TSH falls below 0.4 and by measuring free T3 and free T4 levels.

The Free T3 and Free T4 are used to monitor the treatment. They should be above the median (middle) and below the upper end of the laboratory normal reference range. The goal for healthy young adults would be to have numbers close to the upper part of the range and for cardiac and/or elderly patients, the numbers should be in the middle of its range.

The Free T3 and Free T4 levels should be checked every month and the hormone therapy readjusted until the FT3 and FT4 levels are in the therapeutic range described. Once a therapeutic range is achieved the levels should be checked at least once a year. A small number of large, overweight, thyroid-resistant women may need 6-8 grains of Armour thyroid per day. If you experience nervousness, hot sweats, rapid weight loss, tremor or clammy skin, then the dose should be decreased despite the lab level.

Some patients cannot tolerate Armour thyroid for various reasons and if this is the case you should consider taking cytomel or T3 if you are currently taking Synthroid (thyroxine). In this situation, one may then add 5-12.5 mcg Cytomel (pure-T3) after breakfast and supper daily, rather than Armour Thyroid or Thyrolar (synthetic T4/T3 combo).

Once or twice daily dosing one can then optimize both the T4 and T3 levels, with whatever thyroid preparation is required. This is not possible in most hypothyroid patients with T4 only preparations. Patients with congestive heart failure or severe lung problems may not be the best candidates for Armour because metabolic slowing effect of a low FT3 level can actually be life-saving. However, the vast majority of hypothyroid patients do not have this problem.

Armour Thyroid provides the best results for the majority of patients. Armour thyroid not only contains T3 and T4, but it contains many other factors that facilitate the conversion of T4 to T3 including calcitonin, T1, T2, and many other chemicals. Armour

Thyroid has been around for almost 100 years and has proven to be extremely safe and effective.

A number of factors can contribute to the inability to convert T4 to T3, including:

1. Deficiencies of zinc, selenium, iodine and iron

2. Beta blockers, Dilantin and certain other drugs

3. Alcohol, toxins, synthetic hormones and pesticides

All patients with thyroid problems need to be properly evaluated for vitamin and mineral deficiencies. Just by correcting dietary insufficiencies, thyroid symptoms will usually improve. It is well known that adequate protein and fat is necessary to convert T4 to T3. Excessive iodine supplementation can aggravate some autoimmune thyroid conditions, so you have to be careful with iodine supplementation in these cases.

A deficiency of thyroid hormone can slow down metabolic actions in the body and cause weight gain. Consumption of soy protein can boost the body's natural secretion of thyroid hormone, thereby increasing the body's metabolic rate. Thyroid hormone also is necessary to drive glucose into the cells.

Chapter 6

"Behave or Poop Your Pants"
Tricks of Dietary Fat Absorption Control

Fat around your middle is not only unattractive, but can be down right dangerous because it promotes the release of proinflammatory "cytokines" that seem to be involved in just about every inflammatory process that happens in the body. Even heart disease, strokes, and blood clots are due to inflammatory processes that occur within the lining of the blood vessels. Other inflammatory conditions include cancer and dementia among many others. There is a blood test you can take to measure this effect in your body. It is called a C-reactive protein (CRP). When you have fat that accumulates around your middle abdominal section, a complicated cascade of metabolic processes begin. A term has been coined for this called syndrome x or metabolic syndrome. Most people will have abnormal blood sugars, high cholesterol and elevated CRP.

Dietary fat absorption control is vital to weight loss. There are several ways to accomplish this. The first is not to take in the fat; the other, in a nutshell, is to block the absorption of it once you take it in. It is, of course, hard to avoid that greasy burger sometimes, but you're better off because the latter process is a bit tricky, if not yucky. Using the fat-blocking method alone, however, fails to meet the expectations of most overweight individuals. One reason is that excess carbohydrate absorption will cause the same disruption of metabolic processes, as well as, overconsumption of dietary fats. So, this means drugs that block the rate of carbohydrate absorption may not help ether if you take in too much fat. As we age, the metabolic capacity to efficiently convert ingested calories into energy decreases. Metabolic challenges over time in overweight people accumulate. When you have been overweight for a long time, your metabolism becomes so severely compromised that unless you make corrections in insulin, thyroid, steroid hormones, and feedback hormones, you will never be able to achieve weight loss even in response to calorie restriction. With age and time our cells begin to decline in the ability to correctly utilize resting cellular energy expenditure. This is called a reduction in metabolic rate. This is why you actually may gain weight even when you are eating less. This confirms weight loss is a multi-factorial process. It has been shown that a substance called Irvingia works to block the enzymes that break down sugars and fats and increases your resting metabolic rate. Irvingia contains an alpha-glucosidase inhibitor that reduces up to 90% of postprandial (after a meal) blood glucose spikes and up to 40% decrease in postprandial insulin.

There is a hormone called leptin in our bodies, I discussed under the sleep section. Although leptin injected into rats makes them lose weight, researchers found that doesn't work in humans. Obese people have plenty of leptin. What happens is they become resistant to its affects just like when insulin and blood sugar becomes resistant. Like insulin resistance, leptin resistance leads to chronic inflammatory conditions. Irvingia may correct leptin resistance, promoting weight loss, and combating components of metabolic syndrome. Taking 150 mg twice a day may lead to decreased body fat percentage and waist circumference, decreased cholesterol LDL, C-reactive protein, and fasting glucose.

So how does Irvingia work? It is kinda tricky but it facilitates the breakdown of body fat by reducing an enzyme called glycerol-3-phosphate dehydrogenase that enables glucose to be stored as triglyceride in fat cells. Woo-hoo, and decreases triglyceride levels!!! It also increases the insulin-sensitizing hormone adiponectin and inhibits the digestive enzyme amylase which is involved in carbohydrate digestion.

Some good choices that help leptin resistance include avoiding high-glycemic load and processed foods, supplementing with anti-inflammatory omega-3 essential fatty acids, and engaging in regular

111

physical activity. If you have been overweight a long time, when you do lose weight you cause your body to experience relative leptin insufficiency. The amount of leptin your body requires to stay lean may exceed what your body has when you are thin and all of this causes adaptations to muscle metabolism and modulations in sympathetic and autonomic hormone functions that make weight regain all, but inevitable. Even worse, elevated leptin provokes the growth of certain malignancies, including many forms of breast cancer which helps explain the higher breast cancer risk observed in overweight women.

Adiponectin comes from fat cells and is low when you are overweight. As you lose, weight adiponectin increases and insulin response improves.

Irvingia has also been experimentally shown to inhibit digestive enzymes responsible for breaking down complex carbohydrates into simple sugars. As a result of this activity, it reduces the rate at which glucose enters the bloodstream. This, in turn, lowers the glycemic index of absorbed carbohydrates. Irvingia also reduces appetite by signaling the brain that you are full.

Other ways to block fat absorption include prescription Orlistat which inhibits pancreatic and gastric lipase. It can block up to 30% of ingested fats.

Orlistat inhibits pancreatic and gastric lipase. It decreases the intestinal absorption of fats by 30% by reducing the breakdown of fat. Formerly by prescription, Orlistat is now over the counter in a form called "Alli". Be careful though, if you eat too much fat you might have orange greasy stools, diarrhea or worse stooling accidents... You gotta behave!

Some people overeat too much and have high amounts of fat sitting around for hours after a meal. For some patients, drugs or nutrients inhibit the enzymes that would normally break these fats down will cause gastrointestinal discomforts. You may be best served to only use enzyme inhibitors for a short stent of a month to a few months.

Maybe start with low doses and increase as tolerated. All the while, we must educate ourselves about life-long dietary patterns that will work long term.

The temporary use of compounds that inhibit fat and sugar absorption is designed to "break" the "food addiction" cycle which causes so many people to be overweight or obese. For example, if one's diet consists of more than 30% calories from fat, a lipase inhibitor drug will induce unpleasant gastrointestinal side effects and provide strong motivation for the patient to make healthier food choices. Any patient with a fasting triglyceride blood level over 80 mg/dL should consider Alli and those over 150 mg/dL may also have elevated blood sugar and may want to consider both a sugar blocker and a fat blocker. Inhibiting carbohydrate absorption will help reduce triglyceride and glucose blood levels.

It's no secret; as we age, we no longer have the capacity to consume the same amount of calories we did in our younger years.

Orlistat improves insulin and glucose blood levels and decreased CRP while influencing other blood markers like leptin and adiponectin that are involved with obesity. Due to cost, you might ask your doctor for a prescription of Orlistat as the relatively high cost of over-the-counter "Alli" may be cost prohibitive and patients with insurance coverage might save some money.

As mentioned in the insulin section, chromium and magnesium help insulin resistance. Why do we mention insulin resistance here? Because insulin resistance prevents serum glucose from entering cells and if glucose cannot get into the cells to produce energy, it will be stored in the body as fat.

Chromium picolinate and magnesium have been shown to help break down cellular insulin resistance. For chromium to be effective in the body, niacin must be present. Magnesium deficiency is another cause of excess weight gain in Americans. It is recommended to take one 200 mcg chromium picolinate capsule with niacin/ day, with 500 mg elemental magnesium.

Conjugated linoleic acid (CLA) is a component of beef and milk. It can reduce body fat. It is essential for the transport of dietary fat into cells. Fat not used for anabolic energy production is converted into new fat cells. A deficiency of CLA can inhibit fat from entering muscle cells which can result in excessive accumulation of body fat. It may take up to three weeks to see results, but the protection against magnesium deficiency-induced atherosclerosis, and even a probable reduction in the risk of cancer makes it worth the time invested. The recommended dose is 1000 mg three times a day (best on an empty stomach).

Alphalinoleic acid (ALA) is an essential fatty acid that helps with the metabolism of fat. It is the building block of healthy fats that form the membranes of our cells and signal fat to do work in the membrane and not store in the cell. ALA breaks down into eicosaentaenoic acid (EPA) and docosahexaenoic acid (DHA). Fat is burned as fuel in the cell. To improve the burning or lipolysis, you need fatty acids present to do this.

DMAE is an antioxidant that stimulates nerves and muscles to tighten under the skin and prevents sagging or the not so pretty cellulite.

Coenzyme Q10 is an essential compound required in the proper transport and breakdown of fat into energy.
Clinical studies have shown that CoQ10 may help promote weight loss. In one study coenzyme Q10 levels were found to be low in fifty-two percent of overweight subjects tested. Treatment with 100 mg of CoQ10 was found to accelerate weight loss resulting from a low-calorie diet.
Recommended Dosage: 100-300 mg of CoQ10 per day.

Carnitine helps transport fats in the bloodstream into the mitochondria (where the cellular energy or power produced) for burning. It has the ability to break up tat deposits and aids in weight loss. It also helps to reduce cravings for sweets and fats. Though the body naturally produces carnitine, people who are overweight rarely make enough.

In clinical trials, overweight volunteers taking 200 mcg of chromium picolinate with 100 mg of L- carnitine daily, plus vitamins and minerals, have been shown to average a 15- pound weight loss in eight weeks. Dose: Take 500 milligrams two to three times daily, in conjunction with exercise.

L-Tyrosine suppresses cravings and has antidepressant qualities. It stimulates the thyroid and strengthens metabolic function. Dosage: Take 500 milligrams of L-tyrosine each morning or at bedtime for three weeks.

Gamma Linoleic Acid (GLA) can increase the metabolic rate, an effect that causes the body to burn fat, resulting in weight loss. The average American diet has a deficiency of GLA because of the large amounts of trans fatty acids, sugar, red meats, and dairy products that are consumed. GLA is very difficult to find in the diet, but is found in high amounts in borage, black currant, and evening primrose oils.

Chitosan is an awesome fat binding fiber that binds to fat molecules in the intestines and prevents fat from being absorbed and converted readily into body fat. The recommended dose is three to six 500-mg chitosan capsules and one 1,000-mg ascorbic acid capsule right before a high-fat meal.

You should not take chitosan and CLA together. The chitosan will absorb the CLA. It is best to take your essential fatty acid oil supplements all together first thing in the morning if you are going to use chitosan throughout the day to absorb dietary fat.

There are a few principles to fat metabolism that are vital for you to understand. I read a book called "Outsmarting the Female Fat Cell". It was life changing for me. I still believe you need all the steps in my program to have a fail proof system. If you fail to understand the physiology of fat, you will completely miss the boat. I highly recommend this book by Debra Waterhouse, MPH, RD.

The first premise of the book is you can't starve a fat cell. Meaning, the more you "diet" or try to limit calories too much, the fat cell has a memory and gets smarter each time. Each time you try to lose weight, what you are actually losing is muscle more than fat. Then, when you gain the weight back (as yo-yo dieters always do), then you have lost ground each time because the fat cells get smarter and hang on to the fat better and better each time. It completely explains why each time you diet you lose weight and then you gain back even more than you had before. I love the idea of being able to eat just about anything I want because meal planning is very difficult for me.

One of the hardest issues, I dealt with, was overeating. I would do fine until dinner time and then, although, I wasn't that hungry I found myself binging until my belly felt like a beached whale. One of the things I gleaned from "Outsmarting the Female Fat Cell" was the concept of overeating to be just as dangerous. Overeating may be more dangerous than starving or fasting, as far as, the fat cell is concerned. Debra Waterhouse has a ten step rating scale from very hungry to very full and your goal is to stay somewhere in the middle range at all times. This controls the production and breakdown of fat in the cells and keeps them from outsmarting you. She also emphasizes limiting fats in the diet (because they convert directly to fat) and the need for exercise. Not just any exercise since men and women are different in this regard because of the role that estrogen plays. Women need to exercise for 45 minutes or more, comfortably aerobic (able to sing pace) at least three times a week, to activate the enzymes that break down fat.

So, if you didn't feel like exercise was important before, you need to understand why it has to be a part of an active weight loss and wellness plan especially in women. This book also addresses the reasons we eat and overeat and gives specific steps to control an out of control process.

As mentioned in the thyroid section, deficiency of thyroid hormone can slow down metabolic actions in the body and cause weight gain. Soy protein can boost the body's natural secretion of thyroid hormone, thereby increasing the body's metabolic rate. Thyroid hormone also is necessary to drive glucose into the cells. The isoflavones contained in soy protein extracts have potent cancer-prevention effects, especially against breast and prostate cancer. Soy protein also has been shown to lower cholesterol through its thyroid hormone stimulating effect. It is recommended to take about 20 grams of Soy powder or 5-10 Soy tablets/day.

Hormone deficiencies are a cause of age-associated weight gain. DHEA has been shown to boost insulin growth factor (IGF-1) in humans. The increase may be responsible for the fat reduction and anabolic effects seen in aging individuals. Benefits include immune enhancement, protection against memory loss, reductions in risks of certain cancers, alleviation of depression, and protection against osteoporosis. It is recommended for men to take 50-75 mg a day and women 25-50 mg/day.

Basic supplements needed if you are trying to lose weight:

Chromium 50-200 micrograms (chromium picolinate)
Copper 3 milligrams
Magnesium 250-500 milligrams
Vitamin C 1,000 milligrams
Vitamin E 400 international units
Zinc 15-30 milligrams
Calcium 1,000 milligrams, 1,500 milligrams for postmenopausal women Plus a multivitamin/mineral supplement containing the Daily Values of all essential vitamins and minerals

Summary:

1. Irvigna helps fat metabolism.
2. Orlistat may be used to block the absorption of fat in the gastrointestinal tract.
3. Chromium and magnesium helps with insulin sensitivity and blocks glucose from turning to fat.
4. CLA helps defer fat storage.

5. Chitosan is a great fiber that soaks up fat in the gastrointestinal system and keeps it from being absorbed.
6. Soy may help thyroid metabolism of fat more efficient.
7. DHEA may help with hormone imbalance of fat absorption.

Chapter 7

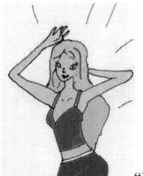

"Let's Get Physical"
Why You Must Increase Your Physical Activity

Increase physical activity. Exercise! Yes, you will have to exercise if you want to consume more calories than you are allowed in a day. No magic fairy dust here. It doesn't mean you have to go out and join a gym or buy expensive equipment. You must find something you can do without causing pain or injury.

You may want to talk to your doctor about options. Almost everybody can walk. You don't need a treadmill, if it is too cold outside. You can walk in your house. Everyone has a little space they can at least pace. There is no excuse. I love my exercise DVDs because I can do them in my living room in my underwear if I want. I like...*Turbo Jam, 10 minute solutions, exercise ball workout for dummies, the wave, and core rhythms...* Most of all, I love my Wii and the "*Just Dance*" programs. They are so much fun and easy to do. Just commit to 20 minutes 3-5 times a week and it will change your life.

Remember, don't eat within 1-2 hours of your workout or you will just burn the calories you consumed, defeating your purpose. You want to burn the "stored stuff". You want your insulin level low and keep it low during the workout. You can drink all the water you want. Watch the sports drinks; they have carbs, unless you are using creatine (more about that later).

Exercise is effective in slowing aging and in helping to prevent heart disease, arthritis, osteoporosis, and other diseases of aging. It also strengthens bones and muscles. Exercise prevents arthritis, most likely, because a well-conditioned muscular system keeps the body in proper alignment. Since muscles hold the skeletal system in place, weak and out-of-shape muscles cause the body to be poorly aligned anatomically. When joints become crowded, their natural gaps and lubrication is reduced, so grinding during movement wears them down even further.

You must be careful not to "over exercise" because if you push beyond your metabolic capabilities you become subject to a variety of ailments including tissue damage hormone imbalance immune system dysfunction or injury. Combined with the use of performance-enhancing drugs, such as anabolic steroids and amphetamines, many athletes are destroying their health in their quest for glory. Exercise must be part of a healthy lifestyle, including a good diet and nutrition. Avoid negative habits, like smoking and excessive alcohol.

Exercise does not have to be vigorous or difficult but requires extra demand on your system which is not normally experienced. Many patients say "Well, I walk all day at work." As I said earlier, with extra demands (not normal experiences) your body will adapt to the new (good) stress and become conditioned, stronger and healthier. This means you should change your exercise routines regularly, as well.

You must exercise correctly and learn how to do it without causing injury. You need to educate yourself and also know your goals. If you perform below your expectations on some days; it is ok. Your body has its own biorhythms and will fluctuate in energy and strength from one day to another.

The biggest thing is to do something you enjoy and just do it.

Remember you're never too old to start exercising. Start now! It doesn't matter how old you are. Exercise can also slow down cognitive or mental decline changes that often accompany aging. Exercise has also been shown to increase learning and memory by doubling the number of cells in a part of the brain called the hippocampus. Exercise has been shown to improve immunity, reduce body fat, and improve mood states. It is a known fact; regular exercise improves glucose metabolism and insulin sensitivity and reduces cholesterol levels.

While exercise is wonderful, there are circumstances when it can do more harm than good. Over-exercising or incorrectly exercising is stressful on the joints and can cause something called oxidative stress. Those who eat poorly, smoke, or do drugs can really increase the risk of oxidative stress while exercising. If you live in areas of high ozone, oxidative stress can be worsened. Taking supplemental antioxidants can reduce this oxidative stress. Whey protein (40 grams) may help as an antioxidant and improve the immune system depleted by exercise under the wrong circumstances by increasing glutathione, the body's most important water soluble antioxidant.

Other supplements that may help regular exercisers are calcium, magnesium, potassium, and boron. Combining them with a good diet is recommended. To maintain healthy joints needed to exercise effectively, you may benefit from nutrients known to improve joint health/function such as:

Glucosamine and Chondroitin - Glucosamine is a precursor for glycosaminoglycans, a major component of the cartilage in joints. It has been found that supplemental glucosamine may help to prevent cartilage degeneration and treat arthritis. Chondroitin sulfate is sometimes used in conjunction and is thought to increase its efficacy. Supporting the joints is essential to healthy exercise and protecting the structure. It is recommended to take 1500 mg/day.

SAMe - SAMe (S-adenosylmethionine) is a molecule all living cells, including our own, produce constantly. Methylation is a process in which molecules donate methyl groups to other molecules.

Methylation occurs a billion times a second throughout the body, affecting everything from fetal development to brain function. It regulates the expression of genes, preserves the fatty membranes that insulate our cells and helps regulate the action of various hormones and neurotransmitters like serotonin, melatonin, dopamine and adrenaline. SAMe is the most active of all methyl donors.

Our bodies need protein to make SAMe from methionine. When SAMe molecule loses its methyl group, it breaks down to form homocysteine which can be toxic if it builds up within cells. B vitamins (B6, B12 and folic acid) help our bodies convert homocysteine into glutathione, a valuable antioxidant that counters this effect. SAMe and homocysteine are essentially two versions of the same molecule: good and bad guys.

When our cells have adequate B vitamins, the brisk pace of methylation keeps homocysteine levels low. When we're low on those vitamins, homocysteine can build up quickly and slow or stop the production of SAMe and cause many problems with our health. High homocysteine is a major risk factor for heart attack and stroke. During pregnancy, it raises the risk of spina bifida and other birth defects. And many studies have implicated it in depression. Elevated homocysteine increases inflammation and counters adequate attempts at the body to burn fat.

Omega-3 fatty acids (fish oil) studies have shown daily fish oil and moderate exercise are enough to influence weight loss even without other dietary changes. The Omega-3 fatty acids in oily fish can contribute to significant weight loss by increasing the elasticity of blood vessel walls and improving the flow of blood to muscles during exercise. Taking a 45-minute walk three times a week appears sufficient to produce the weight loss benefit.

Carnitine - Glycine Propionyl-L-Carnitine (GPLC) is a component of several nutritional supplements that report potent effect of this compound on elevating blood nitric oxide essential to effective exercise. Nitric oxide is responsible for increasing blood flow to active tissues, decreasing free radicals known to interfere with performance and decreasing muscle fatigue. One of carnitines precursors is an amino acid called glycine.

Lipoic acid and creatinine monohydrate - Alpha-lipoic acid has been found to enhance glucose uptake into skeletal muscle. Studies have also found that the co-ingestion of carbohydrate along with creatine increases muscle creatine uptake by a process related to insulin-stimulated glucose disposal. I love creatine. It is one supplement I highly recommend to regular exercisers. It helps maintain higher levels of ATP during exercise and enhances physical performance while minimizing fatigue. What does this mean? You get really awesome muscles when you work out on a regular basis.

Creatine is naturally synthesized in the human body. Approximately 95% of the body's total creatine content is located in skeletal muscle. Creatine is an organic constituent of meat. It has been shown that a more concentrated form of it, taken orally in the form of creatine supplements, may improve athletic performance during brief, intense activities, such as sprints. It is very common among body builders to enhance muscle mass and tone.

I find creatine allows me to load more weight in my workout and be less sore. I hear a lot of patients tell me they are afraid they will bloat or make them too "muscley" or bulky looking. I find my results are incredible and although I did experience some bloating in the beginning it only lasted a few days. The bloating is an overall body bloat. It's not like your typical "monthly bloat". You will carry the water weight in your muscles, so the more muscle you have the more you will notice the water weight. When I am on Creatine, I carry about 3-5 pounds of extra water weight. When you stop it for a few days, the water weight drops very quickly.

"So, what does it do?" you might ask. In a nutshell, it helps your muscles get the nutrients they need to perform, recover, and grow by increasing the blood flow to your muscles causing greater, more effective contractions during your weight-lifting. In addition, it helps your muscles have a continuous supply of the nutrients they need to become leaner and more dense. The best thing about building muscle is that it BURNS FAT!

I recommend taking two to three 3g-5g doses daily in a punch form (high glycemic index juice is needed to create the transport system for the creatine go into your cells). There is no need to "LOAD" this substance, as once recommended. If you choose to load, then the recommended dose is twenty to thirty grams the first 4-7 days, then five to fifteen grams thereafter. The easiest time of day to take it is in the morning and again after your workout. The optional third dose should be taken prior to your workout. You will feel the effects within a week. I recommend taking it for a period of 6-9 weeks and then going off for another 3-6 weeks to check your progress. Then start taking it again for periods of 2-12 weeks at a time, all depending on your goals. I found I had more energy, more muscle stamina, more intense muscle contraction, and better muscle recovery. I was also able to increase my strength gains.

All of these above supplements may prevent age-related mitochondrial exhaustion that intense exercise or over-exercise may do to create free radicals that are especially damaging to the mitochondria in cells.

Ephedrine with caffeine (EC) in small amounts has shown to improve performance prior to exercise by improving fat loss and preserving muscle mass and may have a thermogenic effect. Since EC products are stimulants, anyone with high blood pressure should not use them and always check with your doctor as there are some other medical conditions that are contraindicated, as well. Stimulants can be hard on the adrenal glands, so I am cautious to recommend this to anyone who is at risk for adrenal fatigue or insufficiency.

Challenge equals change! You must constantly be changing and developing your body contour to burn fat and sculpt your image.

Summary:

1. Gotta move it and love it!

2. You can have more calories; if you burn more.

3. Glucosamine and Chondroitin, SAMe, omega-3 fatty acids (fish oil), Lipoic acid creatinine monohydrate and Carnitine may all help you with your exercise regimen, improve oxygenation and protect your joints to prevent over-exercise injury.

4. Challenge equals change! You constantly have to challenge yourself to improve your body contour, tolerance levels and fat burning qualities.

Chapter 8

"If You're Happy and You Know it…"
Normalizing Brain Serotonin

So what is serotonin? It is a neurotransmitter, or chemical that carries messages from the brain, and comes from tryptophan. The most common place serotonin hangs out or has the most receptors are in the brain, of course. It is also found in little known, platelets (clotting elements of the blood) and the gastrointestinal tract. It has been scientifically linked to feelings of well-being; therefore, it is also known as "the happy hormone" (not really a hormone though). Eighty percent of the human body's total serotonin is located in the gastrointestinal system where it is used to regulate intestinal movements. The rest is used in the brain to regulate mood, appetite, sleep, and muscle contraction. It has been linked to memory and learning.

Serotonin is made from the amino acid L-tryptophan. Why do we take tryptophan instead of serotonin? Serotonin taken orally does not pass into the serotonergic pathways of the central nervous system, because it does not cross the blood-brain barrier. Tryptophan and its breakdown products 5-hydroxytrptophan (5-HTP) do. These agents are available as dietary supplements and may be effective as serotonergic agents.

When serotonin is secreted from the gastrointestinal system, it is actively taken up by blood platelets, which store it. When the platelets bind to a clot, they secrete the serotonin; it serves as a vasoconstrictor and helps to regulate the clotting of blood. Serotonin may also help with wound healing, as it is known to be a growth factor for some types of cells. In the liver, serotonin is mainly metabolized to 5-HIAA. After a few metabolic conversions, it is processed by the liver and excreted by the kidneys

So, what has this got to do with weight loss? Serotonin levels are enhanced by carbohydrate ingestion. How does this work? Well, when insulin release accelerates, the blood removes other amino acids that compete for serotonin on the pathway to the brain.

Increasing the serotonin levels in the blood has an appetite suppressing effect. Supplementing with serotonin or tryptophan enhances release of serotonin from the brain and decreases the craving or appetite for carbohydrates, which helps with loss of body weight. Obese people are often insulin-resistant. Diminished insulin action may cause low plasma tryptophan ratios because of the peripheral effects of insulin on the uptake and utilization of other amino acids. If elevation of the tryptophan in relation to the other large amino acids occurs, more tryptophan is allowed into the brain to induce serotonin synthesis, conversion to tryptophan and influence mood, appetite, sleep, and hunger. It is recommended to take 750 mg twice daily and may cause some sleepiness or fatigue. Vitamin B6, magnesium, lysine, niacinamide, curcumin and Vitamin C are needed for the conversion process to tryptophan as well. It has been shown that the higher 1000 mg to 4000 mg is needed for insomnia. Evening, oral doses of tryptophan, as low as 250 mg, have been shown to improve sleep quality. 3500 mg doses may be effective with smoking cessation if the person is also trying to quit smoking, as well as lose weight. 2000 mg a day in divided doses is the best way to saturate the brain fully for most of a 24-hour period for most people. A daily dose of 6,000 mg of L-tryptophan can be used for PMS (premenstrual syndrome) symptoms.

Anti-depressants work mostly by blocking the re-uptake of serotonin in the brain. If you are on an anti-depressant, you need to talk to your doctor first. There is a condition called serotonin syndrome: you get agitated and twitchy when you get too much serotonin. This effect is most risky with MAO-inhibitor medication. There is also a risk of extreme sedation if taken with herbs like St. John's Wort, valarian, and kava kava.

Medications by prescription to restore serotonin or prevent degradation are:

-   Wellbutrin

- Strattera
- Lexapro

Strattera is great to improve your focus and is used often in attention deficit disorders.

Wellbutrin decreases addictive behaviors and decreases stress while attempting to cut calories.

Lexapro can actually cause weight gain in some folks; be careful with this one and use it only if you are mildly to moderately depressed. Eating can be self-treatment for depression. Helping this decreases the need to eat to feel better.

Serotonin is not the only neurochemical at play. It closely regulates dopamine. Dopamine is an excitatory and inhibitory neurotransmitter depending on the dopamine receptor it binds to. It is derived from the amino acid tyrosine. Dopamine is the precursor to norepinephrine and epinephrine, which are all catecholamines. Dopamine plays a large role in the pleasure/reward pathway (addiction and thrills), memory, and motor control. Dopamine, like norepinephrine and epinephrine, is stored in vesicles in the axon terminal (part of the nerve).

Low dopamine levels can cause depression, loss of motor control, loss of satisfaction, addictions, cravings, compulsions, low sex drive, poor attention, lack of motivation and focus. When dopamine levels are elevated, symptoms may manifest in the form of anxiety, paranoia, or hyperactivity.

Other symptoms of dopamine imbalance include: feeling cold or having cold hands or feet, tendency to put on weight too easily, or feel the urge to be motivated by consuming a lot of coffee or other "uppers" like sugar, diet soda, ephedra, or cocaine. Dopamine levels are depleted by stress, certain antidepressants, drug use, poor nutrition, and poor sleep. Alcohol, caffeine, and sugar all seem to decrease dopamine activity in the brain.

There are many natural ways to increase dopamine. Food sources of dopamine increasing tyrosine include almonds, avocados, bananas, dairy products, lima beans, pumpkin seeds, and sesame seeds. Dopamine is easily oxidized. Foods that are rich in antioxidants, such as fruits and vegetables, may help protect dopamine-using neurons from free radical damage. Many healthcare professionals recommend supplementing with vitamin C, vitamin E, and other antioxidants. Foods, such as sugar, saturated fats, cholesterol, and refined foods, interfere with proper brain function and can cause low dopamine.

Caffeine must also be avoided by persons with depression. Caffeine is a stimulant which initially speeds up neurotransmission, raises the amount of serotonin, and temporarily elevates mood. In the long run though, it decreases dopamine and can put stress on the adrenals.

If you need more dopamine and do not eat enough sources of dietary precursors, you can supplement with dopamine precursors that are specific amino acids our brains utilize to manufacture dopamine. Neurotransmitters are frequently not supplied in great enough levels by our modern diet and stress further depletes supplies. 5-HTP, Glutamine, Tyrosine and dl- Phenylalanine with vitamins B6 and C help convert these amino acids into brain dopamine neurotransmitters involved in cravings for carbohydrates, drugs and alcohol, mood and energy levels. They provide balanced serotonin and dopamine support.

If there is anything you learn and practice after reading my book, I would hope it would be from this section. It is so important you take a deep look at your relationship with food and learn to master your food, not vice versa. Otherwise, the information I have provided becomes like every other fad diet. You will go out of balance again and start to gain your weight back.

As I mentioned before, there are so many stressors affecting the hormones in our bodies. This continual pressure on our glands and organs can cause us to act inappropriately as we move, communicate and eat. We have to begin to develop strategies and habits to support the goals we set as we work toward the fabulous person.

I understand and you must understand that the scale is not the most accurate way to tell if you are making the proper changes in your body. I'm not saying to toss your bathroom scale into the garbage. It can still be a useful tool in our toolbox. I have found the most accurate judge of progress is the fit of clothing. As the body begins shifting, you should find you are able to wear smaller dress or pant sizes. These changes may or may not be immediately evident on the scale. In fact, you may actually lose 5 pounds and not see any change in your clothing fit. This can be psychologically damaging to our fabulous goal. Changes to clothing fit, however, tend to be more permanent as we move forward and tend to provide the psychological boost needed. The first long term goal you need to set is the size of clothing you want to "pull off the rack" and put on your body.

What is your relationship with food? How does food make you feel? These are important questions to consider as we move toward the fabulous. Let me suggest you get a pen and paper out right now and start writing. First, write the question "What is my relationship with food?" Take the time to write an honest commentary under this title. Then do the same exercise with the second question.

Consider the following bullet point statements as you write your answers and try to wrench out those statements you tell yourself about your food and your weight. Don't forget to include those food relationships and rituals you experience during the holidays or vacations.

- My parents told me to eat everything on my plate when I was little.
- There are starving children who would love to have my food.
- Being wasteful is a sin.
- I am happiest when eating.
- I am happy, so I eat.
- I am sad, so I eat.

- I am depressed, so I eat to feel better.
- Eating a big breakfast is smart.
- Eating a big dinner helps me sleep.
- I only eat one meal a day.
- It's the holiday season.
- I'm just going to have to start dieting tomorrow.
- My body craves certain foods.
- I eat lots of meat to help me build muscle.
- I would rather eat than have sex.
- When I look in the mirror, all I see is fat.
- My scale is way off.
- Beer is healthy.
- A sip of alcohol before bedtime helps me sleep.
- I gain weight even when I eat hardly anything.
- I'm pretty sure I have a thyroid problem.
- Being overweight is genetic for me.
- Smoking helps keep me thin.
- Addicts are weak.
- Bacon makes everything taste better.
- I'm pregnant; so I can eat whatever I want.
- Chocolate makes everything taste better.

Keep your dialogue in a safe place and we'll come back and review it. Remember to be honest with yourself. If it helps you to be honest, hide these documents in a safe place and show them to no one. It is extremely important you are able to review your heart-felt feelings about your food habits and rituals on a day-to-day basis and your food issues during vacation or holidays.

THE BLESSING OF ABUNDANCE OFTEN LEADS TO THE CURSE OF INDULGENCE

I was watching a documentary recently about the events surrounding the assassination of President Kennedy in the early 1960s. As I watched the terrible events unfold in Dallas, I was side-struck by how thin the people in the crowds appeared. I thought about general population and crowds I have been around recently and how obese we look compared to fifty years ago. This begs the question, "What has changed so drastically in our society that we are so obese today?"

Let's discuss one of the ugly things that might be a cause for this: cigarettes. As a physician, it is incumbent upon me to speak of the terrible disease and heartache that comes from smoking cigarettes. Studies do show, however, that there is a substantial risk of developing type II diabetes for folks who quit smoking. That does not mean I would ever suggest anyone keep smoking, in order, to avoid getting fat.

One thing that is not reported often is that alcoholics who make the commitment to quit drinking are also prone to gain weight. What is the underlying cause for this trend toward obesity for those who give up such terrible habits?

Our society accepts that smoking and alcoholism are terrible, addictive habits. However, not much is said about the terrible, addictive habit of overeating. For now, food seems to be off the list of things we should be avoiding for our body's health; even though, we all know being obese is bad for you. Let's be honest and admit it is not the fault of food that we are obese. Perhaps instead, we should consider how our society is terribly undereducated about the development of addictive qualities and how to avoid them.

Consider a recent report on how teenagers were becoming highly addicted to texting with their mobile phones. My interpretation of this report suggested this addiction among teens was overtaking the cigarette as the addiction of choice. There didn't seem to be a great deal of concern in the report about the psychological nature of addiction development. One should wonder: if a teen were to be banned from their cell phone for a week, would they turn to food for comfort?

One more ugly addiction is sex addiction. As a physician, I see patients who are swingers or sex addicts. In almost every instance, these folks are overweight. Apparently, one addiction tends to lead to another; especially if one is denied. Finding help for the addict inside is essential. I am suggesting most people who are overweight today may have developed an addictive personality.

For many, the idea of addiction conjures up images of junkies lying on the sidewalks with needle tracks and blown out veins all over their bodies or the drunk staggering down the street barely able to keep their footing. The truth is there are many addicts among us. There are those addicted to making money, playing video games, collecting garbage or other things…the list goes on and on. Whatever the addiction, there is a strong psychological attachment that is extremely difficult to break, which is why addiction support groups or counseling are a must.

I do prefer to use the term addiction when speaking of things others may wish to refer to as bad habits. The term addiction implies there is a morbid condition that goes beyond a simple habit. Although there are habits we might consider good, like exercising, we are less likely to refer to these a "good addictions." We have to keep in mind, good habits like exercise are easy to fall out of which is not the case with addictions. Addictions require acknowledgment and acceptance of its existence and that we will have to live with it the rest of our lives.

THE FACE(S) IN THE MIRROR

Who is it that you see when you look in the mirror? Do you see a beautiful child of God, pure in spirit, elegantly and masterfully designed? Or do you see the ugly fat person, the cheater, the loser, the liar or thief? Self-perception is key to your decision making progress as you move throughout your day.

Consider, for a moment, the spiral effect the addict inflicts upon themselves through their decision making progress.

The object of affection presents itself to the addict. It is at this point a critical decision takes place, either by the self or the addict within. When the addict is allowed to choose, the addict will always choose the object or event that brings the immediate pleasure. The addict knows they are in control and the addict knows the pleasure is guaranteed. So the addict commits the act.

If the self still exists, it realizes that it has given the power over to the addict. So, the self is now inflicted with guilt. You may not realize this, but the addict thrives on the self's admission of guilt. Guilt absolutely empowers the addict to take more and more control until eventually it drives the self completely out of the body. That's why I began this paragraph with "if the self still exists."

This is why you see the advancement of addiction leading to families being torn apart and careers thrown away. As the addict assumes more control, it trusts and chooses the objects or events it is able to control. People are not easily controlled and are too unpredictable for the addicts taste. The addict wants simply to experience controlled pleasure at all cost.

At this point, let me emphasize the importance of releasing yourself from guilt, especially if you think you see the addict in you. You absolutely should acknowledge your bad choices, but at the same time consider the correct choices. Again, self-loathing will only empower the addict within and allow opportunity for reemergence.

I was recently attending class with my first grader and was impressed with what his teacher was doing to raise student awareness of their choices. When a child acted out she would say "That is a bad choice. What is a better choice?" and the child had an opportunity to be empowered by positive choices. This kind of thought process can work for you, as well. Set out to retrain your mind to make correct choices. As we work to develop this in our minds, it becomes a good habit we can carry with us and serves to ward off the reemergence of the addict within.

EATING TO PREVENT WASTE ULTIMATELY LEADS TO INCREASED WAIST

The fabulous person understands the title of this section. You know, we could spend hours discussing the merits of certain diets like all protein or all carbohydrate diets. People have written books about it, for goodness sake, and we have spent our money supporting these theories. When it comes down to it, however, the simplest thing you should be doing is counting your calories. It's so simple: calories IN = calories OUT. Why make it more complicated than that?

An excellent resource I recommend is myfitnesspal.com. On this website, you can track your intake of calories and your caloric use in exercise. There have been many contributors to the caloric database; so, you are almost guaranteed success as you begin to track your calories. The learning curve is a little steep in the beginning as you become to take note of calorie content, consumption, and . Remember, why you eat is as important to understand as what you eat.

ARE YOU FABULOUS???

What is holding you back?

What is holding you back from making the changes you need to make in your life?

"If you always do what you have always done, then you will always get what you always got!"

If your life or health is not what you want it to be then you and only you can change it! You can't keep doing the same thing you've always done and expect it to change.

Healing, wellness and feeling fabulous is a journey. To be the fabulous you that you deserve to be you must make true change in your life. You must start your journey. You must embrace change.

Two things hold us back from making change: "Fear" and "Lack of Trust"
To embrace change you may have to face your fears.

Fear can be protective, but what about when it keeps you from living the life you dream. What can you do about fear? How can you overcome it?

What are you afraid of?

Do this exercise! It will change your life.
Write down on a piece of paper all the things you are afraid of. List them one by one. It can be a short list or long, but be honest. Then burn the list. Place it in a tin can with a glass of water near by and watch the paper slowly burn. Take a deep breath and let the ritual engulf you. Let it go. Let it all go! This is the first step. Then use the tips that follow to live your life in love and trust—NOT FEAR!

1. Face your fear to become stronger. SERIOUSLY? Or not?
Don't take your fear so seriously. You might think to yourself that what you thought was a fear before wasn't that much to be afraid of at all. Everything is relative. And every triumph, problem, fear and experience becomes bigger or smaller depending to what you compare it to.
But to gain a wider perspective of human experience and grow you really have to step up and face your fear.

2. Take action and get busy.
"Inaction breeds doubt and fear. Action breeds confidence and courage. If you want to conquer fear, do not sit home and think about it. Go out and get busy." Dale Carnegie
Waiting and worrying about the fear helps nothing. Rally your troops. Get input from others. Make contact with the fear. Get in it's face.

"Worry gives a small thing a big shadow."Swedish proverb
99% of the things we worry about happening, never happen and 99% of the things that happen, that we should have worried about, we never thought of.

3. Focus on Love

When you hold others and make physical contact a hormone called oxtocin is released in the brain. This is the love hormone that helps moms to be affectionate and cuddle their babies. It is thought to be deficient in those with anxiety disorders and those with focus disorders or chronic pain, all physical manifestations of fear and lack of trust.

Here are ways to naturally boost your body's oxytocin production:

Hugs-Just embracing others, holding hands, or draping an arm around your significant other, child, or person you care for can produce an increase in oxytocin.

Make eye contact-When you interact with others oxytocin can be enhanced with mental embrace as well as physical contact.

Passion-Adults seeking an oxytocin surge should head for the bedroom. The hugging and touching during foreplay fires up the love chemical, and orgasm spikes the hormone level to two times the normal amount. This opens the door to a relaxed feeling and a greater opportunity to bond with your partner.

Get your hormones balanced-Interestingly, among premenopausal women, oxytocin is naturally higher during ovulation because estrogen intensifies the love hormone. This may partially explain why women seem to be more prone to touch and other displays of affection during ovulation.

Daydream-Research out of the University of North Carolina at Chapel Hill discovered that happily married women quickly released a dose of oxytocin when asked to think about their husbands.

Get a pet- A loyal pet is there to make owners feel good and because the release of oxytocin is triggered by touch, petting a dog or cat you love can also increase oxytocin levels.

Get comfortable-Remember the smell of your mother's cookies, hearing kind words from someone you care about, telling someone how much you appreciate them, take a walk with a loved one—these are all ways to boost oxytocin.

You can also get oxytocin supplements if you have severe anxiety or fear issues.

4. Fear is often based on false interpretation or miscommunication. As humans, it is our nature to look for patterns. The problem is just that we often find negative and not so helpful patterns in our lives based on just one or two experiences. Or by misjudging situations. Or through some silly miscommunication. Our brains make neuronal connections to past events. It is important not to judge past experience on future interactions. Every situation is different. We transfer a lot of fear and misgivings into future situations that we should really approach with a fresh perspective.

5. Don't cling to your illusion of safety. The only thing permanent is change and there is no "comfort zone".
One big reason why people don't face their fears is because they think they are safe where they are right now. But the truth is safety is only a sense, like fear, it is not real only perceived. There is no safety out there really. It is all uncertain and unknown.
Life happens, you may lose your job, your loved one, have to move, lose your home or suffer unknown tragedy. You may get laid off. You will eventually die. Who knows what will happen?
This perception of safety is not always a bad thing. It's protective. But there is also not that much point in clinging to an illusion of safety. So you need to find balance where you don't obsessed by the uncertainty but also recognize that it is there and live accordingly. As you stop clinging to your safety life also becomes a whole lot more exciting and interesting. You are no longer as confined by an illusion and realize that you set your limits for what you can do and to a large extent create your own freedom in the world. You are no longer building walls to keep yourself safe as those walls wouldn't protect you anyway.

6. Be curious.
"Curiosity will conquer fear even more than bravery will." James

Stephens
When you are stuck in fear you are closed up. You tend to create division in your world and mind. You create barriers between you and other things/people.
How do you become more curious? One way is to remember how life has become more fun in the past thanks to your curiosity and to remember all the cool things it helped to discover and experience. And then to work at it. Curiosity is a habit. The more curious you are the more curious you become. And over time it becomes more of a natural part of you.

7. Trust the antidote to fear.

 Most of our fears are based on how others perceive us.
The ego wants to divide your world. It wants to create barriers, separation and loves to play the comparison game. The game where people are different compare to you, the game where you are better than someone and worse than someone else. All of that creates fear. Doing the opposite removes fear.

But one thought you may want to try for a day is that everyone you meet is your friend. To take this one step further assume that every one you meet has something to teach you.

There is often an underlying frame of mind in interactions. Either it asks us how we are different to this person. Or how we are the same as this person. This creates warmth, an openness and curiosity within. There is no place to focus on fear or judgment anymore.

This is of course not easy, especially if you have held the first frame of mind for many years. But you can get insight into this by doing the rest of the things above. As you face your fears the barriers and separation you have built in your mind decreases. You come closer and feel more of a connection to other people.

With action, curiousness and understanding we come closer to each other. We gain a greater understanding of ourselves and others. And so it becomes easier to see them in you. And you in them.

Make your change. Don't hold on to your illness and your fear. Start the journey to a new you today! A fabulous YOU.

More about Oxytocin

Oxytocin, a peptide that functions as both a hormone and neurotransmitter, has broad influences on social and emotional processing throughout the brain and body. It has many implications with both weight loss and wellness. Oxytocin's role in reproductive functions is well known. In 1906, the English researcher Sir Henry Dale discovered a substance in the pituitary gland that could speed up the birthing process. He named it oxytocin from the Greek words for quick and child labor. Later, he found that it also promoted the expulsion of breast milk.

Now it appears that oxytocin plays a much larger physiological role than previously recognized, since under many circumstances, it has the ability to produce the effects that we associate with the state of calm and emotional wellbeing or connectedness.

Oxyticin is thought to be the yang of corisol the stress hormone. Everyone needs oxytocin. Everyones body was designed to release Oxytocin. Some of us have experienced stress and trauma to the point that our bodys natural ability to create oxytocin is depleted. Nearly everyone experiences stress to a degree.

Love is the feeling and experience that ties us together. When we experience too much stress and anxiety in our lives, it breaks down vital relationships and leaves us feeling lonely and isolated. Adults who are under constant stress and anxiety experience more bouts of depression, dissatisfaction in life and increased health challenges.

In humans, oxytocin is released during hugging and pleasant physical touch. It plays a part in the human sexual response cycle. It appears to change the brain signals related to social recognition via facial expressions, perhaps by changing the firing of the amygdala, the part of the brain that plays a primary role in the processing of important emotional stimuli. In this way, oxytocin in the brain may be a potent mediator of human social behavior.

In 1998 a study by Kovac was done that showed that Oxytocin reduced food cravings and sugar cravings, calms the mood and produces satiety sensations through counteracting stress.

As stated before here are a few natural ways to increase your oxytocin:

Share a warm hug or a kiss
Cuddle
Make love
Sing
Get or give a massage
Hold a baby, a dog or cat
Perform a generous act
Pray or meditate
Show support

Oxytocin plays a vital role in promoting factors that enhance well-being. Oxytocin plays a critical role at enhancing factors within the individual which promote well-being. Oxytocin induces increase in level of trust and reduction of fear through modulating the response of amygdala and other central structures to stress and fear. Oxytocin increases approach and pro-social behavior and enhances social interactions, as evidenced by human and animal studies. Oxytocin reduces subjective sense of anxiety, increases overall calm and is implicated in non-verbal intelligence.

Summary:

1. A healthy serotonin level is vital to proper metabolism.
2. Serotonin can be increased by natural means by supplementing with tryptophan, the oral precursor to serotonin.

3. Prescription medications may keep serotonin around longer.
4. Serotonin deficiency leads to obesity through many mechanisms, including signaling of satiety.
5. Serotonin interacts with many other neurochemicals, like dopamine, to signal appropriate eating and overeating habits.
6. Why you eat is as important as what you eat.
7. Oxytocin is vital to wellbeing and balancing cortisol

Chapter 9

"Burn, Baby, Burn"
Improving Energy Expenditure Rate

To lose weight, you have to burn fat. Everybody knows this. "Why is it so important?" you might ask. Well, as we age there is a significant decrease in resting energy expenditure.

One of the easiest ways to burn fat is to use a diet pill. Stimulants are best known for increasing resting energy expenditure and suppressing the appetite. Some of the medications are by prescription and are Phentermine, Adipex, and Bontril.

Other Options include:

[] *Fucoxanthin* and *pomegranate seed oil* - Fucoxanthin is a substance found in plants. It is a xanthophyll or pigment in brown algae. Some metabolic and nutritional studies carried out on rats and mice at Hokkaido University indicate that fucoxanthin promotes fat burning within fat cells of white fat/adipose tissue by increasing the expression of something called thermogenin. A study in obese women showed an average 4.9 kg (11 lb) weight loss over a 16-week period It is not a stimulant like ephedrine.

[] Green tea polyphenol – Researchers suggest if the average person were to drink five cups of green tea a day, they would burn an extra 70 to 80 extra calories through an effect known as thermogenesis. Some of the effect is from caffeine.

[] *Fish oils* rich in EPA and DHA -- These omega-3 fatty acids help with thermogenesis (fat burning). They inhibit key enzymes responsible for lipid synthesis, such as fatty acid synthase and stearoyl-CoA desaturase-1, enhance lipid oxidation and fat burning, and inhibit free fatty acids from entering adipocytes (fat cells) for fat storage.

[] *Conjugated linoleic acid,* in particular the *trans*-10, *cis*-12 isomer has metabolic benefits that include increased energy expenditure, decreased fat cell differentiation and proliferation, decreased fat synthesis, and increased fat burning and fat oxidation.

[] *Capsaicin,* the active agent in red pepper - Capsaicin can decrease appetite. During a study, 24 men and women were given about ½ a teaspoon of red pepper, close to .9 g of the red pepper which contains 0.25% capsaicin, thirty minutes before every meal. Other members of the study were given a placebo without their knowledge. After eating their meal, the subjects' saity increased when they were given the red pepper and less calories and fat were consumed. Those who took the placebo had minimal change in saity compared to saity after a meal when they didn't take the placebo.

The study also found in post-consumption, more energy was expended by those involved in the test. Capsaicin creates these results by increasing thermogenesis (the body burning energy from food released as heat), "enhancing catecholamine secretion from the adrenal medulla". The increase in thermogenesis suggests a change in "substrate oxidation from carbohydrate to fat oxidation". These amazing outcomes say capsaicin increases fat burning and weight loss almost seem too good to be true! The results are legitimate and strong, but like all new research, multiple studies should be done to test the consistency.

[] Extracts of *ginger* rich in *gingerols* and *shogaols* - Shagaol also known as (6)-shogaol is a pungent constituent of ginger similar to gingerol. It is produced when ginger is dried or cooked. Shogaols are artifacts formed during storage or through excess heat, probably created by a dehydration reaction of the gingerols. The ratio of shogaols to gingerols sometimes is taken as an indication of product quality. It is moderately more pungent than piperine, but less than capsaicin, and has similar effects to capsaicin in thermogenisis.

Chapter 10

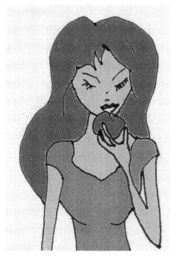

"It's Gotta Stick!"
Adopting a Long-term Healthy Eating Strategy

J.P. is a patient of mine who has been seeing me for almost seven months. He is morbidly obese and trying to make changes. I recently told him that his diabetes, high blood pressure, congestive heart failure and fatty liver which lead to cirrhosis and liver failure had become critical and he was essentially dying. Despite this, his health continued to decline. Before he started my program, he continued to overeat. Even when faced with life-threatening diseases related to their obesity, most overweight people simply cannot manage to eat less.

One overlooked reason for today's obesity epidemic is a stress-induced disorder known as "emotional eating." Consuming certain foods, especially high-glycemic carbohydrates, bolsters "feel-good" brain neurotransmitters such as serotonin, often depleted by stress.

Increasing brain serotonin levels through high-carbohydrate meals can help elevate mood in the short-term. This behavior long-term is dangerous because it leads to weight gain. To stand any chance of

145

success, programs designed to help people reach and maintain an optimal body weight must address the multifaceted biochemical and psychological processes that contribute to excess weight gain. The key is to understand the intricate interplay of messages that suppress brain chemicals and trigger the urge to overeat, activating hormones that convey to the brain a sense of satiety and fullness, and optimize metabolic processes that contribute to increased fat burning and lean body mass.

It's happened to everyone. Most of the time, we are able to successfully control our food intake. We balance our caloric intake with our daily caloric expenditure in a way that prevents weight gain. Then the inevitable "stress event" kicks in and we head for the "bad stuff". Emotional eating is a way many people cope with negative feelings like depression, anxiety, stress, and boredom.

The chemistry of emotional eating is a complicated. One way of explaining it is that eating more carbs or sugars than proteins allows more of an amino acid called tryptophan into the brain to convert to serotonin and relieve stress by stimulating the release of brain opioids, known as endorphins. Endorphins are the feel good stuff. Soon you feel pleasure and then dopamine, another neurotransmitter, triggers a positive reward system that triggers the anticipation of pleasure each time you repeat this cycle. Other hormones are imbalanced by this tipping of the scale, such as cholecystokinin (CCK), glucagon-like peptide-1 (GLP-1), leptin, and peptide YY, which also influence hunger levels. Successful manipulation of these neurotransmitters, hormones, and peptides can therefore help prevent episodes of emotional or stress eating.

Green oat extract - Avena sativa (green oats) works by freeing up testosterone that gets bound to various compounds or proteins in the body. Protein bound testosterone is not as effective as free testosterone and along with stimulating growth hormone provides fertile ground for muscle growth. A study done in 2008, from the Department of General Surgery at Baskent University in Ankara, Turkey, found the wild, green oat extract Neuravena increased the delta and theta brain waves associated with the brain regions closely connected to mental performance. In addition, Aydogan confirmed the intake of Neuravena had positive effects on cognitive function and helps increase overall mental fitness in an individual's life. Green oat extract may help ease emotional stress and nervous energy by increasing the action of two chemical messengers that enhance positive feelings. Laboratory studies have found wild oat extract significantly inhibits two enzymes that are closely related to mood states: monoamine oxidase B (MAO-B) and phosphodiesterase-4 (PDE4). MAO-B is responsible for the breakdown of dopamine. Drugs that lessen its activity are frequently used to treat symptoms of depression. Inhibiting PDE4, on the other hand, helps to boost levels of cyclic AMP (cAMP), an important secondary chemical messenger in cells, thereby promoting the positive feelings that can decrease emotional eating.

Pinolenic acid – from Korean pine nut oil helps with specific reactions in the body that suppress appetite cravings in the brain. When we eat, the intestines release satiety hormones, such as cholecystokinin (CCK) and glucagon-like peptide-1 (GLP-1). These circulating hormones convey information about food intake and appetite to the brain pathways to tell us we are full. Pine nut oil can dramatically increase CCK and GLP-1 levels.

Conjugated Linolenic Acid (CLA) - Studies suggest that CLA is effective for a number of reasons and has been shown to reduce fat uptake into the adipocytes (fat cells). This effect is thought to promote an increased flux of fatty acids to the muscle cells, boosting the use of fat for fuel. The result would be a sparing of liver glycogen stores, which researchers believe may contribute to satiety signals. CLA-induced changes in gene expression promote apoptosis (cell death) in the adipocytes, helping to reduce the number of cells that can store fatty acids.

No fad diets ever again!!! Make healthy choices and you'll never go wrong.

Must haves… water and vitamins!

Drink lots of water. Sometimes your body thinks you are hungry and you are really thirsty. Sometimes the stomach gets used to the large expansion from large portion sizes and big meals, so if you drink a lot of water, especially, before you start eating, your stomach will think it is fuller than it is. The hydration, also, helps mobilize fat stores and increases your metabolism. Once you get used to reducing your portion sizes, you will be amazed at how much fuller you feel faster. It takes a few days to kick in, but your body really does learn to adapt to your schedule and your intake

Take a multivitamin! Ideally you should eat healthy proportions, but this is not always ideal with our busy schedules. It doesn't really matter what brand, although some are better quality than others. I recommend a lot of different supplements, but the basic multivitamin will get you at baseline where you need to be.

You can use the info at www.myfitnesspal.com to calculate your individual needs for proteins, carbs, fat, and vitamins based on the foods you eat. This takes all the guess work out!

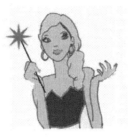

What would you do if you had a magic wand?

What would you change about your world????

How many times have I heard, "If only I had a magic wand..."

And sometimes when I meet patients that have so many health concerns that they need to address and reverse, I ask them. "If I had a magic wand and could change one thing for you today.... what would it be?"

This gives us a starting point for making changes.

Most patients I meet would like to change something about themselves. Most of them seem to have lost the ability to believe that they have the power to change.

So often we get frustrated by what I call the "Vicious Health Cycle". We start by making unhealthy choices. Then we find ourselves feeling guilty about those choices and then overindulging in more unhealthy behaviors until it looks like there is no turning back.

When I give my patients a "magic wand", I remind them that it is REAL! I tell them that it only has the power that they give it and remind them of the 3 rules.

1. Use it only for good - This is because when you empower yourself to make changes you only want positive changes and these are the only changes that will really impact your life and health. If you wish ill on others you are only damaging your own psyche, not conducive to healing and making positive changes in your own life. Think of ill will towards others as a big sack on your back. Each person that makes you angry or has wronged you is a potato in that sack. If you carry that sack around for a week or two what happens? It begins to rot and stink. Others smell the odor and you feel sick from the nauseating aroma. You add a few more potatoes (or folks who have wronged you) and soon you have a bad back from carrying all that weight. Your adrenal glands mimic this sack on your back. They carry all the stress of anger and regret. Even one rotten stinky potato is enough to cause serious damage to your health. Make a commitment today to drop the sack!

2. Magic takes time - Once you believe and the changes start to happen, you must have the faith to keep the "vicious health cycle" from spiraling out of control again. Patience is so difficult to have in our "instant gratification" society. When you start to see results patience becomes easier. To have good health and see positive changes you have to educate yourself about the processes in your body and how to take control of out of control cycles. You can't beat yourself up about slip ups and mistakes. You learn from them, recognize your triggers and redirect. Knowing that you have the magic power to move forward will keep the goal real and the focus in site.

3. Believe - A dear friend gave me a little sign that I keep in my bathroom by my make-up mirror. It reads, "She believed she could - so she did". It's really that simple. When you seek out the answers to changing your health and becoming the most fabulous YOU, that you can be you really do start to believe.

Believe! Believe! Believe!

You can do anything you desire. You can reverse disease and find health. All you have to do is BELIEVE and COMMIT!

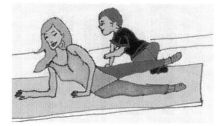

Avoid negativity! Even those who love you may discourage you at first. When my son was five, he would pull at me during exercise when I first started and say "Mommy, I'm hungry. Mommy I need you." He wanted me to do this or that, always something. When he got the idea exercise was important to me, he backed off. He had no underlying motive other than my attention. Then, there are the hidden agendas. Spouses or significant others who may be jealous of your success, that you may be attractive to others if you achieve your goal, or just apprehensive to change. Finding rice cakes and celery, instead of cookies or doughnuts, may be frustrating to them if they are not on board with you. We eat not because we are hungry, but often for entertainment, stress, boredom, sleepiness or other reasons. You must get adequate sleep to balance your hormones (including the hunger regulating hormones). Your insulin levels and your moods need stabilizing. You will get easily frustrated and discouraged if you are tired and fussy. Make your goals known and stick to them. Anticipate the negativity you will get from others. Embrace it and consider it all part of the challenge.

Don't become nutrient deficient when attempting to lose weight
The biggest mistake people make when trying to lose weight is reducing their nutritional intake as they reduce their caloric intake. This is a critical mistake.

When working to lose weight, you must greatly increase the

nutritional density of your diet so you're getting MORE nutrition with FEWER calories. You've got to drop the junk foods, filler foods and processed foods and turn to high-density superfoods and nutritional supplements that can nourish your body even while you're consuming fewer calories.

This is the big secret to weight loss that's entirely missed by most celebrities, infomercials and even many weight loss coaches: Eat MORE superfoods, drink MORE water, and take MORE supplements. Only when your body is fully nourished with nutrients and minerals will it be willing to safely let go of body fat.

A word about cravings:
While you're thinking about controlling your appetite, you might ask yourself: Why do I have cravings in the first place?

Most people who have cravings for carbs or sugar (or even snack foods) are chronically deficient in trace minerals. One way to get your minerals is to take a trace mineral supplement or eat Celtic Sea Salt, Royal Himalayan Salt, or other various "natural" salts.

There is a reality about weight loss people need to be aware of. Losing weight requires you to feel hungry from time to time. There is no way to lose weight without feeling some degree of hunger. Believe me, I have exhaustively explored this issue. I have tried appetite suppressants. I have tried food combinations. I have tried meal-timing strategies. I have tried just about everything natural under the sun to eliminate those hunger pains and food cravings you get when you are attempting to lose weight. There is nothing that completely eliminates those cravings. And honestly, you wouldn't want to shut your body's ability to be hungry. It is essential to life.

The key is to understand and empower yourself to know what to do when the call of your chemicals comes and realize there is nothing wrong with hunger and it is a normal human response to a decrease in your consumption of calories. The problem most people encounter when they feel hungry is they feel it's some sort of emergency or urgency, like they are dying or wasting away. In fact, the body is

152

just signaling it doesn't have enough calories to add new fat to the fat stores it's already carrying around. Embrace these feelings and know what they are telling you.

Here comes the first wave. A little ping in the pit of your stomach. A quiet rumble. The first feelings of hunger are really more of a false alarm than anything to be concerned about. This is your primitive brain response to consume calories: "Where are the chips?"

But, wait. STOP. Before the next wave of hunger hits, let your frontal lobe kick in and know what to do.

The first thing you need to do is have an arsenal of foods ready that you can instinctually run to so you don't have to think a lot about your choices. The primitive brain may ruin your change of eating something healthy or making wise choices. You need to have foods you can turn to when you are feeling intense hunger pains, but you don't want to add significant calories to your daily intake.

I call these "Impulse Solutions."

Impulse Solution #1

H2O!!! Water. That's right: water is a powerful appetite suppressant and if you drink an 8-ounce glass of water when you first start feeling hungry, you will find it suppresses your appetite in nearly every case. If you drink just one full glass of water and have the discipline to wait 10 minutes, you will find your appetite is either completely gone or dramatically reduced.

Impulse Solution #2

Warm organic chicken or vegetable broth. Avoid those with MSG, yeast extract, autolyzed yeast extract, hydrolyzed vegetable proteins, and other similar ingredients with heavy salt, as they can stimulate hunger. Only 20 calories and you can completely fill up.

Impulse Solution #3

Green vegetables such as lettuce, cabbage, or bokchoy among many. You can allow yourself to eat an unlimited quantity of any green leafy vegetables without even recording the number of calories in your log without guilt. I love FREE calorie food! Its free calorie food because it takes just as many calories for your body to digest as you get out of the foods themselves. And yet at the same time, they fill your stomach and make you feel full, turning off the hunger signals in your brain.

Best way... fill up a very large bowl with lettuce and salad greens, then add only 100 calories worth of dressing. You will want to find some of the lower calorie salad dressings out there, and of course you want to avoid MSG, high-fructose corn syrup, and other ingredients in salad dressings. You can also stir fry them in a pan by using water and flavoring like onions, garlic, and soy sauce. Stir fry all the green vegetables you want. They count for zero calories.

Impulse Solution #4

Smoothies, shakes and puddings! Low calorie solution: Add a quart of soy milk to the blender, then a couple of scoops of unsweetened banana-flavored simply natural spirutein soy powder. Add splenda or stevia powder as a sweetener if needed. And you have a smoothie or shake. To really add some appetite suppressant qualities, while the blender is running, put in about 1/2 tablespoon of guar gum powder, plus another 1/2 tablespoon of xanthan gum powder as thickeners. The whole mixture will attain the consistency of pudding. Now just pour it into a bowl and eat it like banana pudding!

Impulse Solution #5

Natural pickles or apples. Not the pickles you find at a regular grocery store with artificial preservatives or colors. Apples are great for appetite suppressants because the bulky fiber fills up your stomach and turns off your appetite control hormones before you overeat. Plus, apples contain various phytonutrients, vitamins, and minerals.

Impulse Solution #6

Fiber tablets. Take psyllium husk, glucomannan, oat bran fiber, apple pectin fiber, or other natural fibers before you begin eating. Drink plenty of water as you take these pills because without adequate water they can obstruct your digestive tract. By consuming both the fiber and the water before you start eating, you've already significantly turned off your appetite. Then by consuming these extremely low caloric density foods and beverages, you will further suppress your appetite. You can get an entire meal into your stomach for 100 calories or less and you can trick your brain into thinking you consumed an all-you-can-eat buffet.

But there's a catch to all this: in about an hour or so, your body will figure out there isn't much energy in the food you've consumed. Your hunger will begin to return, but at least you delayed the onset of that hunger by an hour or more. If you combine this with physical exercise, you can delay it even further because the very act of exercising releases stored body fat and converts it back into blood sugar, which raises your blood sugar level and suppresses your appetite cravings. You can also extend the effect of this by taking appetite suppressant supplements like phentermine (by prescription) or Hoodia, but only during your "jump start" phase of weight loss as these can be stressful to your adrenal glands long term.

Also, you don't want to starve yourself by eating these impulse foods all day long. Remember, starvation is the fastest way to train your body to hold on to body fat. These are just items to get you past a difficult time when your appetite is unbearably intense. Each day, you still need to get nutrition into your body in the form of whole foods and whole food supplements.

Overall, keep in mind that achieving your healthy weigh loss goals takes effort. You will experience moments of intense hunger and these low-calorie, filling foods are one excellent way to get through a difficult time without packing on the pounds.

Final Word: Tips and secrets!

- Avoid salt. It makes you more hungry, as do artificial sweeteners and MSG.
- Avoid TV. Take a TV fast. Do housework, vacuum, call a friend and pace while you talk.
- If it's not worth the calories, don't eat it.
- Don't starve yourself.
- Don't skip meals.
- Take pride in your appearance.
- AVOID people who have motive to keep you fat.
- Don't be too hard on yourself.
- Don't exercise after eating, you just burn the meal.
- Keep track of your calories and limit them to less than 1200 / day.

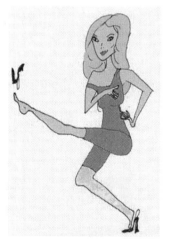

Beauty Secrets: How to look young forever....

Drink LOTS of water and avoid sodas like the plaque as the sodium dehydrates you and depletes your bones and skin of valuable nutrients.

Retin-A-Micro daily on face and neck.

Bio-dyne Canadian 50 G Preparation H Ointment with Bio-dyne large 50 gram size. Bio-dyne, a natural yeast cell extract, is the models' secret for younger looking eyes.

Botox to prevent static lines from forming from dynamic lines, as well as, to treat current wrinkles.

Bio-oil daily on decollage area (neck).

Microdermabrasion and chemical peels regularly.

IPL skin re-surfacing for sun damage.

Juvaderm to plump lips for that pouty look.

Radiesse for scars or old acne spots, deep wrinkles or dimples.

Exilis for cellulite or creams that contain caffeine.

Vitamin C, 4000 mg a day for age spots on the skin and those who bruise easy.

Biotin for hair and nails.

Thyroid support for healthy glow.

Plenty of testosterone to make you feel "sexy".

Coconut or Moroccon oil for dry hair ends.

Rev up your exercise with hand and ankle weights and get an indoor exercise trampoline to increase your aerobic burn and maximize calorie expenditure.

Use sunless tanners (I love Banana Boat TM sunless tanner) and never tan your face, but get plenty of sun (without burning) to increase your Vitamin D.

Bio-identical hormone cream will keep you skin elastic and supple.

Dry cracked heels use "Kerasal" for one step exfoliating and moisturizing. Use "Callus-eliminator" from "Be Natural" and rough grade sandpaper, if really flaky.

I wish you all the best! Health and Happiness! I wish you the ability to run and play with your children without getting short of breath. Freedom from joint pain from carrying around too much weight. Increased self-esteem and the power of knowing you can do this. Beauty to sustain you INSIDE and OUT!

You have the secrets now. Not just the idea but the actual tools.

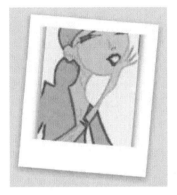

My Favorite Meal Plans:

No special diets! Eat what you want but here's what to focus on:

Eat only when you feel your "stomach" not your head, tell you are hungry usually this hits every 3 hours.

Water: LOTS!! Drink 1-2 gallons/ day.

Rule of thumb: when the hunger hits:
    1. Drink an 8 oz. glass of water.
    2. Wait 10 min. to see if those pains persist.
    3. If so, simply eat. If not, wait until the pains return and then eat.

Protein: remember each gram of protein has 4 calories. At least 600 calories a day of a 1200 calorie diet should come from protein. Eat your goal body weight in protein grams/day.

Carbohydrates: limit these as much as possible. That is between 3-4 servings of carbs a day. Plenty for your energy and nutritional needs.

Fat: at least 30% fat should be your goal. You may want to cut almost all the fat out of your diet to lose weight. You need fat for satiety and sanity. If you have a meal with no fat, you will be hungry again within 2 hours. By adding a little more fat, that meal will keep you satisfied for 3-4 hours. Everything in moderation!

Greens:
Green veggies or lower carb veggies. They are so low in calories, you can eat until you're full! So eat your greens.

Treats:
Eat only your goal weight in calories for a treat. If you want to way 125 then only eat 125 calories worth of that huge piece of decadent chocolate cake. You can enjoy the 125 calories worth!!!!
My Favorite Exercises!

Aerobics: Wii-Just Dance 1 and 2, Wii-Zumba, Swimming, Walking, Dancing

Exercise Ball: Sit ups and crunches

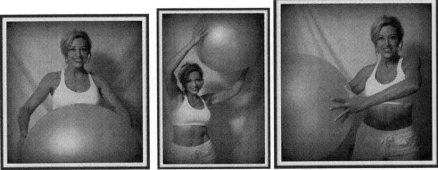

Exercise Ball: Round the world
Start with your exercise ball above your head, arms extended then rotate the ball clockwise for 5 reps then counterclockwise for 5 reps. A stay ball with sand in it really works your arms. Suck in your abs while you do this exercise for more ab work.

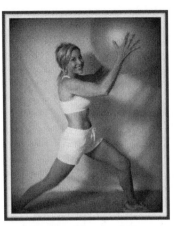

Lunges
Stand with ball in front of you and lunge forward then pull the ball
into your extended knee and repeat 11 reps.

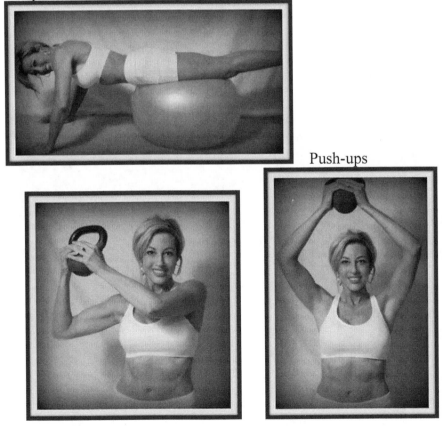

Push-ups

160

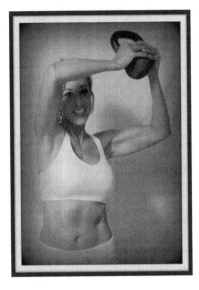 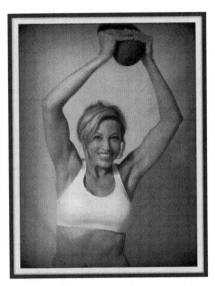

Kettle Bell: Round the world
Same things as with the ball but now with a heavier weight. Start with 3lb. kettle bell. Never lift more than you can handle with muscle fatigue.

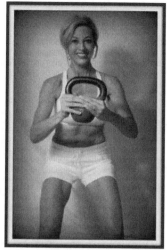

Ski bumps
Hold kettle bell in front and
bend knees, like you are going
Over little bumps skiing.

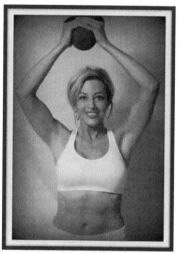

Hula-hoop
Hold kettle bell overhead
and rotate hips like you
Are doing a hula-hoop.

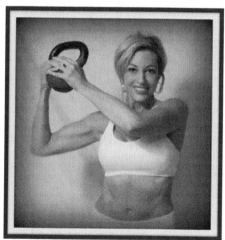

Throws
Kettle bell up over shoulder and
drop down to opposite knee.
Drops

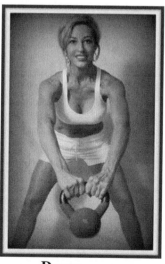

Drops
Kettle bell throws into
the middle of the inner
thighs and back out.

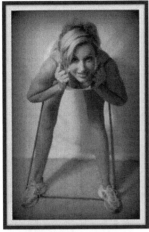

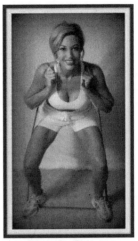

Band: Froggies

Band: Squats

Bend over with the Band around your
Shoulders and feet. Keep your abs
Vertical with the floor and bend your
Knees. 11 reps

Squat all the way down
to your knees buttocks to
ankles. 11 reps

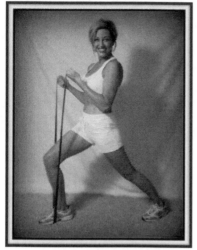
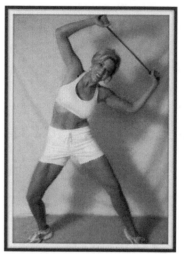

Band: Lunges
Band stretched out, lunge
deep bending back leg.
bends. 11 reps

Band: Side Bends
Use band to stretch side
side to side overhead.
11 reps

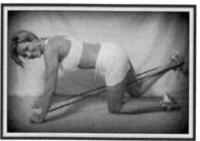

Band: Donkey Kicks
Stretch band behind and kick out
behind. 11 reps

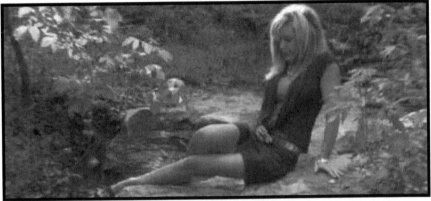

ABOUT THE AUTHOR

Dr. Tammy has spent many years cultivating a culture of accountability in patients. She has motivated and mentored many in the ways of improving their own health one healthy decision at a time. Born and raised in a small town in Arkansas and pursuing her training all throughout the U.S., she is grounded and in tune with the simple to the sophisticated when it comes to educating her patients. Her extensive work and educational background lends to her non-traditional physician approach. She went beyond attaining a bachelor's degree in biology to pursing her master's degree in public health. While doing this, she began teaching and discovered a passion for educating as a means to spawn greatness and discovery in others. She then attended 4 years of medical school at Kansas City University of Medicine and Biosciences plus an additional year at Truman Medical Center as a Pathology fellow teaching and learning about the basics of human processes. Her goal was to integrate all these experiences, so she could be the best family physician and health educator/mentor possible. She did her residency in Tallahassee, Florida. She is currently a board certified family practice physician licensed to practice in the State of Arkansas.

She has done award-winning research in multiple areas including education, cancer, and biologic hormone processes. She has focused additional emphasis on programs promoting wellness and preventive care. She offers her patients a unique approach to medicine by bringing an extensive education, a desire to help others, and a genuine desire to make the medical experience a positive one for all patients. Oh, and she brings a BIG SMILE! Those who know her will confirm she loves enlightening, educating, and empowering others to pursue healthy lifestyles. She has spent the past few years transforming into everything she recommends. She definitely practices what she preaches!